D1597599

Dx + Rx
A Physician's Guide to Medical Writing

Dx+Rx

A Physician's Guide to Medical Writing

John H. Dirckx, M.D.
Medical Director
Student Health Center
University of Dayton
Dayton, Ohio

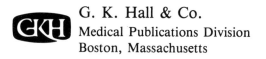
G. K. Hall & Co.
Medical Publications Division
Boston, Massachusetts

To my parents

Contents

Preface

The purpose of this book is to give specific and concrete advice to the physician who wants to improve the accuracy, clarity and readability of his medical writing. Though conceived as a guide for those who write but seldom for publication, it should prove useful also to professional writers, editors, translators and abstracters.

The medical practitioner, teacher or researcher who is called to authorship by inclination or duty may discover that his professional training and experience have ill prepared him for this line of work. Finding himself unequal to the task of presenting his ideas in concise, exact, graceful prose, he naturally looks for help from a manual or textbook of technical writing. I believe that the present volume comes closer to meeting his needs than any other currently available.

The typical manual of technical exposition informs the aspiring author how to arrange graphs, photographs and paragraphs, but does not tell him what to do with words (or, for that matter, what not to do with them). From such broad subjects as the general organization of material and the use of statistics and illustrations, it descends abruptly to the minutiae of punctuation and capitalization, measurements and units, abbreviations and bibliographic form. Meanwhile, the essence of writing —the construction of sentences—is slighted if not altogether omitted. Textbooks of English composition, of course, devote much space to grammar and the mechanics of style, but they do not address the special concerns of the medical writer.

In this book I have tried to deal fully and practically with the real problems that confront the inexperienced writer who undertakes to prepare a technical paper, monograph or book chapter. This is neither a cookbook nor an editorial style manual: it is meant to be read, not merely consulted. I have made no attempt to define or codify standard forms for abbreviations, symbols, units or bibliographic entries, which vary widely from one journal or book publisher to another. To ensure that his work conforms to his publisher's standards a writer must consult and follow that publisher's style manual.

Part I, which will seem superfluous to the reader with a deadline to meet, has the practical purpose of bringing down to earth the airy abstractions of the grammarian and the linguist. Part II is a systematic and mainly positive treatment of the principles according to which logical, forceful, streamlined and appealing technical prose is written. In Part III I have presented a fuller discussion of the "pathology" of writing than is usually thought worthwhile in books on composition. I have not followed the usual practice of manufacturing imaginary or theoretical errors: most of my specimens of faulty writing have appeared in print before.

When a stage magician falls on hard times he sits down and writes a book revealing the secrets of—other magicians. When a writer's well-springs of inspiration dry up, he produces a manual of English composition, dwelling with particular relish on other writers' mistakes. H. L. Mencken once observed that most books on prose style are the work of writers quite unable to write. By the time you arrive at the final chapters of the present volume you may be finding more matter for correction in my text than in my specimen errors. Should this be so, the book will at least have served its purpose of instilling in the reader a spirit of sternly rational criticism toward every sentence of expository prose committed to paper. Of course, in your zeal for unearthing ambiguities, absurdities and stylistic blemishes, you must not forget to turn the spotlight on your own work—preferably before submitting it to an editor for publication.

Dx + Rx
A Physician's Guide to Medical Writing

I

Words: The Anatomy of Language

Aseptic technique is just an irksome and meaningless ritual to one who has no knowledge of microbiology. Similarly, the rules of spelling, punctuation and grammar may seem unduly stringent, if not altogether frivolous, until one understands something of their rationale. I offer this opening section of the book on the nature and purpose of language, and the norms and standards that govern its use, as a foundation and point of departure for the material to follow. It is not, however, essential to an understanding of that material, and the reader may pass over these first two chapters without impairing the practical utility of the other ten.

1

Symbol, Syntax and Sense

Before we can talk about using the English language to best effect we must define language. Though it is easy enough to frame a definition of language as "interpersonal communication through articulate speech or some representation of it," the language thus characterized is an abstraction. We speak and write not language but *a* language, and that is not so easily pinned down.

We might start by calling a language a set of words shared by the members of a race or nation. This concept of a language as a mere vocabulary, superficial and imperfect though it is, gives us an opportunity to focus our attention briefly on words before going on to more intricate subjects.

Only with difficulty can we imagine performing any deep or sustained thinking without using words. In thinking, as in speech and writing, we manipulate ideas and relationships by embodying them in words. In one primitive language the verb for *think* means literally "to talk inside one's belly." Yet no one should really need to talk to himself in order to think. Words, after all, emanate from the tongue, teeth, lips, palate and vocal cords. If man lacked this apparatus his cerebral cortex would surely never have generated so much as a syllable. Words are preeminently vehicles for conveying ideas from one person to another.

Words carry information in two ways. First, each symbolizes or represents some thing, action, quality or relation. In the dawn of human history, language probably went no further than that, each word functioning as a mere isolated label. It is important to note that most words have a range of meanings: there are more things than nouns, more acts than verbs, more qualities than adjectives. Compare the differing senses of

3

human in *human subjects, human blood, human lice.* Contrast the meanings of *for* in "Chloral hydrate was prescribed for sleep" and "Chloral hydrate was prescribed for insomnia."

The literal or primary meaning of a word (on which lexicographers do not always agree) is its denotation. For example, the denotation of hand is "the prehensile organ at the end of the arm." The many derived senses in which the word can be used are its connotations (or its extension): the hands of a clock, a ranch hand, a hand of cards, a hand in the preparations, an old hand, a neat hand, a helping hand, a hand of applause and so on.

To the linguist any indivisible unit of meaning is a morpheme. *I, John, cut, through, liver, non-, neur-, -itis, -plast* and *'s* are all morphemes, at least when regarded as words or parts of words in English, though *-itis* and *-plast* could be broken down further from the viewpoint of Greek grammar. Whereas the first five morphemes in the list can each stand alone, the rest cannot. Independent words are known as free morphemes; prefixes, suffixes and stems as bound morphemes.

Teachers and students of modern languages have the bad habit of confusing *stem* and *root*. A root is a primitive structural unit common to several words in various related languages. The Indo-European root *dhe-*, referring to birth and rearing, has a prodigious offspring in modern English, including *thel-* (= *nipple*), *female, fetus, femur, fecund, felicity* and *filial*. A stem is the part of a particular word that is left when all inflectional material has been taken away. (Though I have not yet defined inflectional material, the following examples should supply several broad hints.) The stem of *breaking* is *break;* of *longest, long;* of *needles, needle;* of *Charley's, Charley.* A survey of the stems of several Latin and Greek words (*sinus, sinu-; astragalus, astragal-; thrix, trich-; iris, irid-*) uncovers a bewildering lack of consistency, which is explained in part by the observation that the term *stem* (like *root*) has historical as well as structural implications.

Eons before the invention of writing, man began forming sentences to express relations between two or more concepts: "I killed a boar," "The fire is out." This second and more advanced way of passing on information with words provides us with a more precise means of defining a language, since no two languages make sentences in exactly the same way.

The arrangement of words in meaningful groups is called syntax. It is only when we look at the role or function of a word in a specific sentence that we can classify it as one of the parts of speech—noun, verb, adjective and the rest. In English the chief clues to the function of a word come from its position: word order makes all the difference between a pocket watch and a watch pocket, between "The man caught the shark" and "The shark caught the man," between "The cock crowing, hope revives" and "The crowing cock revives hope."

A language whose meaning depends on the sequence of words in a sentence is called analytic or isolating. In Chinese, which is strictly analytic, words undergo no change in form, and no word has a fixed role. Whereas in English we can add things to the stem *red* to signal changes in its meaning or function (*redder, redness, redden, reddening*), in Chinese these changes would be shown solely by the position of the word in a sentence, and the word itself would remain unchanged.

Since English can and does alter words to show differences in meaning or relation, it cannot be called purely analytic. Further examples of such change in English are *kidney* → *kidneys, see* → *saw* and *Addison* → *Addison's*. Many of these changes, which are known as flections or inflections, consist in the attachment to the stem of primitive word fragments whose origins were forgotten before men could write. Languages that make extensive use of these imbedded or engrafted word fragments (for example, classical Latin and Greek, and Anglo-Saxon, the ancestor of modern English) are called synthetic.

Most languages are neither purely analytic nor purely synthetic but, like English, somewhere between the extremes. Though German inflects all nouns, adjectives and verbs, it has a far more rigid word order than English. By contrast, the richly inflected classical languages could dispense altogether with word order as a syntactic device.

Even when we put the grammar of a language alongside its dictionary, we are still a long way from defining it. Language is much more than just a means of conveying information: it is the most intricate and sophisticated form of self-expression yet evolved by the human race. Language is behavior. The egotist, the humbug and the prude reveal themselves as plainly by the manner or style of their speech and writing as by its semantic content. Just as manners and morals, costume and cuisine reflect ethnic traits, a language mirrors the attitudes and qualities common to its speakers. Each language is saturated with traces of the country and the culture that produced it. A desert people can get along with a single word for *river, lake* and *ocean,* and may see no need to distinguish *swimming, sailing* and *rowing.* On the other hand, Arabic is said to have 5,744 words referring to the camel. It is no exaggeration to state that the very foundation of Western philosophy, the logic of Aristotle, derived its structure from Western man's modes of predication, that is, his way of talking.

The influence of custom and convention is even more evident in the way in which we suit our level or style of expression to the station and character of the one to whom we are speaking, and his relation to us. The languages in which one addresses his wife, his colleagues, his children, his neighbors' children, his patients, his stockbroker and his garage mechanic all differ in grammar, intonation and phrasing, but most noticeably in choice of words.

We can see similar forces at work in the labeling of some words as polite, others as informal, jocular, pretentious or obscene. Being our most concentrated symbols of thought, words can carry an astounding burden of emotion as well. For proof of this we need only consider the impact of derogatory epithets like *nigger* and *honky,* of proper names like *Benedict Arnold* and *Casanova,* even of abstractions like *evolution* and *Communism.* The physician early learns the dark and potent magic of *malignant, immature* and *venereal.* The jubilant cry of Xenophon's returning troops when they reached the sea, "Thallatta, thalatta," has echoed down the millennia with undamped fervor and an undiminished capacity to thrill the hearer or reader. Julius Caesar's "Veni, vidi, vici" sums up the whole history and personality of the man: the egomania of a Hitler, the military genius of a Napoleon, the nobility of an Alexander. We may with perfect truth turn around the Chinese proverb and say, "One word is worth three thousand pictures."

CHANGE AMID UNIFORMITY

Although a language, in its very essence, is a set of fixed conventions, the one unvarying property of language is incessant change. Let us view some of the ways in which a language grows and evolves before we consider the norms and standards that have been erected as bastions against undesirable change.

So intricate and inscrutable a mystery is the origin of language that in 1866 the French Society of Linguistics formally banned further research on the subject. Many theories, some ingenious and some absurd, have been advanced to explain how language began. It seems probable that talking is no more a deliberate invention than running or laughing. Though a word has no necessary relation to what it represents, neither is it altogether arbitrary: it must somehow correspond to the idea in the mind of the wordmaker.

Many words, for example, owe their origin to onomatopoeia, that is, they echo the sound of what they represent: *borborygmus, click, fremitus, murmur, singultus, stridor.* Though only a fraction of the words in the dictionary are plainly onomatopoetic, it is possible to draw up for each simple consonant cluster a list of native English words which are rather closely related in meaning:

slip, slap, slop, sled, slide, sleigh, slick, slack, slime;

snout, snore, snort, snarl, snicker, sneer, snoop, sniff, snuff, sniffle,
sneeze, snot;

spring, sprig, spray, spread, sprawl, sprout, spout, spit, spatter,
sputter, spark

Few Biblical scholars now insist upon a literal interpretation of the
story of the origin of language in the second chapter of Genesis, or that
of its diversification in the eleventh chapter. The notion that all human
languages evolved from a single parent tongue is inherently improbable.
Still, we have solid evidence that most of the three thousand languages
and dialects presently spoken in the world are descended from a few
primitive systems of speech. The lexical similarities within the great
group of languages that includes the Germanic family (to which English
belongs), the Romance (French, Spanish, Italian and others derived from
Latin), the Indic and the Slavic, suffice to show that these are all derived
from the same primitive tongue, which is known as Indo-European or
Aryan. The patient who says that he has *broken* his *elbow* is really using
the same words as the doctor who prefers to say that he has *fractured* his
olecranon: Anglo-Saxon *brecan* and Latin *frangere* both evolved from
the onomatopoetic Indo-European root *bhreg-,* while Anglo-Saxon
elnboga and Greek *olecranon* (and for that matter Latin *ulna*) had a
common origin from the root *ele- = bend.*

It would be hard to overestimate the role of word-borrowing in the
development of modern Western languages. A borrowing, also called a
loan-word (though the lender continues in possession of it and the
borrower never gives it back) must be distinguished from a legacy or
hand-me-down. At some time after the ninth century the Anglo-Saxons
borrowed *skin* (*skinn*) and *die* (*deya*) from the Danes, adopting them in
favor of their own *hyd* and *steorfan,* which, however, survive in *hide* and
starve. By contrast, they did not borrow *heorte = heart* and *blod = blood*
from any alien tongue, having inherited them from Old Teutonic *herton*
and *blodom,* which in turn sprang from the Indo-European roots *kerd-*
(cf. Latin *cor,* Greek *kardia*) and *bhel-.* English borrowed *fontanel* from
French and *influenza* from Italian, but those languages had inherited
them from their common ancestor Latin.

A language is a process, not a product. Each successive revision of the
dictionary is a fossil before it reaches the printer. Even a "dead"
language like Sanskrit or Latin can be described or studied only within a
temporal frame of reference. The classical Latin scholar has a new
language to learn when he takes up a medieval text, and yet another if he
wants to read Dante in the original.

As a language matures and evolves, its words undergo continual alteration in both form and meaning. Generations of tongues round off sharp corners by a kind of phonetic erosion. Since each ethnic group has its own tastes in sound, shifts in both vowels and consonants tend to follow regular patterns. The elucidation of this natural phenomenon by Grimm and Bopp in the nineteenth century laid the foundation for the modern science of linguistics. Typical vowel changes are seen in the metamorphosis of Latin *os = bone* into Spanish *hueso,* of *dens = tooth* into *diente* and of *umbilicus* into *ombligo.* Consonant changes in Indo-European languages follow a pattern described by Grimm's Law, according to which the *f* of *fracture,* a Latin-derived word, corresponds to *b* in the Germanic *break.*

Some words grow by accretion as they get older and pass from one language to another. The primitive root *ok- = eye* swelled to *ophthalmos* in Greek and gained a diminutive suffix in Latin *oculus.* Latin *cor* appears as *corazón* in Spanish. *Stomachus* and *species* lose their Latin terminations in French but gain introductory syllables: *estomac, espèce.*

Phonetic changes that follow no law or pattern are known to the linguist by the derogatory name of corruptions. When medieval Latin *ischiadicus,* from Greek *ischion = hip,* had lost its first letter and suffered other lesser disfigurements, it emerged as *sciaticus.* Even further from home is *licorice,* originally Greek *glykyrrhiza = sweet root.* We need not chase words from one language to another to find corruptions and other phonetic shifts. In English the passage of a few years often brings about a nearly universal change in the form of a word. The first *r* of *February* is going the way of the first *d* in *Wednesday.* The *p* of *cupboard* and the *th* of *clothes* have not been heard from for decades. Our usual pronunciation of *comfortable* transposes the *t* and the *r,* and we usually put the *r* before the *v* at the end of the French loan *hors d'oeuvre.* Even some cultivated speakers seem to prefer *intregal* and *nucular* to the more conventional and historical pronunciations. As instances of accretion we may point to the extra consonants in the popular mispronunciations *equiptment* and *drownded.*

These examples illustrate the fact that although English spelling is phonetic it lags decades and centuries behind the actual sounds. Fortunately, crusaders for spelling reform are invariably squelched by persons with enough intelligence and foresight to see that any radical change in our spelling would render all our books illegible in a generation. A significant number of spelling corruptions are not of phonetic origin. The fledgling anatomist who has just learned that *hallux* means *the great toe* may be at a loss to understand the etymology of *hallucination.* Medieval Latin *hallucinari* and *hallux* are both purely orthographic corruptions, the original words, *alucinari = to wander in mind* and *allex = thumb,* being unrelated. The presently accepted spellings *antibrachial* and *distention* are corruptions of the earlier and classically correct *antebrachial* and *distension.*

Another important class of change in words is the breakdown, over long periods of time, of grammatical and inflectional distinctions. Clearly there was a time when it seemed important to distinguish *shall* from *will, who* from *whom;* otherwise such distinctions would never have arisen. Just as clearly, *shall* and *whom* are now viewed as superfluous, and are drifting out of style and out of the language.

Semantic change plays an even more vital role in the evolution of a language than phonetic change. A shift in the meaning of a word comes about most often through metaphorical extension, which allows us to speak of an airplane that *lands* on the water, or of the *sailing* date of a steamship. Some china is made in Japan, and, according to the song, "A blackberry's red when it's green." Abstract ideas are commonly labeled with concrete words applied metaphorically. Thus, in most languages words meaning *be* originally denoted some physical act, such as *breathe* or *stand.* A mere inspection of many abstract words shows their origin in the realm of the concrete: *discover, inclination, understand.*

The denotation of a word may gradually shift away from its literal meaning under the influence of its associations. Three muscles arising from the fibula are called *peroneus* (*peroneal*), from *perone,* the Greek name for this bone. The two larger muscles, peroneus longus and peroneus brevis, the principal evertors of the foot, have given the adjective *peroneal* to the lateral muscular compartment of the leg and associated nerves and vessels. Though the peroneus tertius also arises from the fibula, it is not so much an evertor as an extensor of the foot. It lies in the anterior compartment of the leg and is regarded by some as a part of the extensor digitorum longus. Herein lies the basis of the curious statement, found in anatomy textbooks, that "the peroneus tertius is not a peroneal muscle." The literal meaning of peroneal, "pertaining to the fibula," has yielded to an associative meaning, "everting the foot."

An abstract term may lose its literal or historical significance as new information reshapes the concept for which it stands. Thus, obvious misnomers like *detoxication* (not concerned solely with poisons), *gonorrhea* (not "a flow of semen"), *myo-edema* (not edema) and *vitamin* (some are not amines) survive against all odds. Cases of mononucleosis are reported in which the peripheral blood smear is normal, and eponymic terms like Addison's, Graves' or Hodgkin's disease are applied to conditions that do not fulfill the criteria laid down by the original describers. Names of physical phenomena and of diagnostic or therapeutic procedures may also come to mean something quite different than when they were first proposed. Kussmaul's term *pulsus paradoxus* referred to a palpable radial pulse in the absence of cardiac apical impulses during inspiration. The maneuver described by Valsalva for testing or restoring the patency of the auditory (eustachian) tubes was obviously not straining to exhale against the closed glottis, but rather blowing out the cheeks with lips and nostrils compressed.

Convention generally plays at least as important a role as etymology in determining the meaning of a technical term. Both thrombi and fat globules, if released into the venous circulation, will travel to the lungs, yet the phenomena of their arrival there are somewhat irrationally distinguished as *pulmonary embolism* and *fat embolism*. Edema of the optic disc (papilla) is *papilledema* only when it is not due to papillitis!

The meaning or function of a word may also be altered by deliberate fusion with other morphemes through composition (or compounding) and derivation (or affixation). Composition is the coupling of two or more stems, of either native material (*breakdown*), borrowed material (*macrophage*) or a blend (*beeturia*). Affixation refers to the attachment of a prefix (*non-, pre-*) or a suffix (*-hood, -itis*) or both to a stem to form such derivatives as *nonreactive, prerenal, fatherhood* and *colitis*.

Though I have discussed the phonetics of words as distinct from their semantics, form and meaning cannot be dissociated in practice, since each exerts a continuing influence on the other. An interesting example of this interaction is false or folk etymology, as illustrated in *tornado*. Though the original Spanish word *tronada* meant *thunderstorm,* folk etymology has so steadfastly persisted in deriving the corrupted form from *tornar = to turn* that its official meaning in meteorology is now "a whirlwind or storm characterized by spinning air currents," and it never refers to thunder.

False etymology has been responsible for some persistent misunderstandings of medical terms, as when *apocrine* (from Greek *apokrinein = to separate*) is mistakenly thought to refer to the apex of a secretory cell, and *claudication* (from Latin *claudicare = to limp*) is erroneously derived from *claudere = to close up.* "Jaw claudication" and "claudication at bedrest," ludicrous when taken literally, betray an inaccurate notion of vascular pathophysiology even when interpreted in the light of false etymology.

The underlying error in false etymology is the fallacy of false analogy. The patient who takes his friend's medicine because it was prescribed for an ailment similar to his own is "reasoning," probably to a false conclusion, by analogy. For users of English, good spelling demands a continual struggle against the siren charm of analogy. If *siege,* why not *sieze?* If *wield,* why not *wierd?* Why not *sheopard* or *lepherd?* If *Albert, Robert, Hubert* and *Herbert,* why not *sherbert?*

False analogy also explains, and sometimes nearly justifies, grammatical errors like "Nobody was home but Aunt Maggie and I" and "She is older than me." Such errors are even commoner with words taken from the classical languages, whose grammars are closed books to the modern physician. Thus, though *prodromata* seems like a correct plural if one argues from the analogy of *neuromata* and *atheromata, prodroma* is already plural. *Abruptio placenta* may look right alongside *placenta praevia,* but the analogy is false.

The recurring role of false analogy in language error is scarcely an accident, for analogy is one of the dominant forces that shape and hold together a language. New words are built by analogy with old ones: *heliport, motel, skyjack.* Indeed, analogy generates whole families of new words—*-terias* and *-oramas, -urias* and *-ectomies*—and even new usages.

The influence of analogy is nowhere more evident than in the view of a language as a set of substitution frames. For any given sentence we can imagine an unlimited number of other sentences differing from the first by a single word.

> Fredricks *prepared* the solution.
> Fredricks *stirred* the solution.
> Fredricks *boiled* the solution.
> Fredricks *spilled* the solution.
> Fredricks *drank* the solution.

When we hear one of these sentences for the first time we understand it instantly because we perceive it as being analogous to many other similar sentences. Even if a nonsense word is substituted ("Fredricks *zackled* the solution") we still know that Fredricks did something to the solution, and that what he did is represented by *zackled,* a verb in the past tense.

We may think of word families as substitution frames, too. Except for *drank* in the above series, all of the past-tense verbs are of the form *—ed.* Many words of the form *—ly* are adverbs, and nearly all of the form *—ous* are adjectives. The frames *hyper—osis* and *over—ness* may be thought of as synonymous.

When we say that *peroneal* and *Valsalva maneuver* owe their current meanings to their associations, we recognize the operation of analogy under a slightly different guise. The exchange of a primitive meaning for another derived from more recent associations occurs as readily with bound morphemes as with free ones. Thus, *-osis* was a suffix used by the ancient Greeks to convert a verb into the corresponding noun, as in *diagnosis.* Its modern significance, as in *toxoplasmosis,* arose by analogy with the many uses in which it refers to infestations, intoxications or excesses. Similarly, *sternebra* combines the stem of *sternum* with a suffix borrowed from *vertebra* and taken to mean "one of a series of bones."

In classical Latin *-bra,* like Greek *-osis,* is just a suffix for turning a verb into a noun: *vertebra = turning point,* from *vertere.*

UNIFORMITY AMID CHANGE

We take it for granted that two persons who have never had any previous communication can immediately enter upon a discussion of the most abstract and intricate subjects, provided that they speak the same language. Should we be surprised if two persons who have known each other intimately for many years occasionally have difficulty in communicating? Though language draws its form and pattern directly from the operations of the mind, its "logic" is the logic of one who already knows something. This kind of logic does not necessarily enable the speaker to choose his words and construct his sentences in such a way that another mind, however attentive and acute, can grasp his ideas with facility and accuracy.

Transmitting information in writing is an even more delicate and risky procedure. Reflect that, except for numerals and punctuation marks, all the characters printed on this page are symbols for sounds. Of course, not all of the sounds are heard in modern English, and most of the symbols can represent more than one sound. But since letters are phonetic signs, not ideograms, the written word is twice removed from the writer's thought. Small wonder if it sometimes fails to generate in the mind of the reader an accurate replica of that thought. Enter the grammarian.

The first grammarians concerned themselves only with written language, as the word *grammar,* from Greek *graphein = to write,* might suggest. Early Hebrew and Christian philologists had no other purpose in studying and fixing linguistic conventions than Biblical exegesis and the comparison and correction of variant texts of Holy Scripture and of primitive theological writings. Presumably these early grammarians appreciated the elementary fact that spoken and written language are never identical, their vocabularies and syntaxes overlapping only partly.

Spoken English, for example, contains many words and usages that are not yet tolerated in formal writing, and may never be: *lotsa* (*lots of*), *real = very, sure = yes, not really = no, through = finished.* Though the written language preserves the auxiliary verbs *have, must, will* and *wish,* the spoken language has largely replaced them with *yoosta* (*used to*), *sposta* (*supposed to*), *gonna* (*going to*) and *wanna* (*want to*). The written language also has terms and conventions peculiar to itself. No one but a political orator or a pedant says *that of, to whom, deem, esteem, possess, profess, perceive, deceive.*

Syntax is looser in speech than in writing. Repetition and circumlocution are the rule, with accent and gesture taking the place of careful phrasing. Meanings are approximate rather than exact. Though simple words of broad connotation tend to be overworked, nonce words and other unconventional forms also abound. It is easy to misinterpret these differences and fall into the delusion that spoken language is a degenerate, corrupt, imperfect form of the language.

Surely nothing could be plainer than that the spoken language is the language itself, and the written merely a highly sophisticated elaboration of it. The written language, being susceptible of preservation, changes much more slowly than the spoken, retaining conventions and usages that are decades, even centuries out of fashion in speech. Until recently dictionaries either refused to recognize usages peculiar to speech or dismissed them with such scornful labels as "colloquialism" or "dialectal variant."

Modern grammar, in contrast to classical, concerns itself with the spoken language as well as the written. The task of analyzing and codifying the spoken language is fraught with peril, and many of the brightest minds that have undertaken it have succumbed to one fallacy or another. The popular image of the grammarian as a finicky, narrow-minded fanatic no doubt arose from the failure of early students of spoken English to remember that they were describing a natural phenomenon, not the invention of some still earlier grammarian. As Seneca put it two thousand years ago, "Grammarians are the guardians, not the authors, of language."

We owe to Otto Jespersen, indisputably the greatest of English grammarians (though he was Danish), the handy distinction between the descriptive and the prescriptive grammarian. The descriptive grammarian seeks to comprehend the patterns, the order, the system and the consistency of language. His prescriptive confrere turns these patterns into legislation for the guidance of those who wish to speak and write correctly. The prescriptive grammarian is a very useful creature as long as he confines himself to driving errors out of individuals, but when he begins to see errors in the language itself, and to fulminate in priggish indignation against them, his utility ceases and he becomes ridiculous.

The work of the grammarian who undertakes to redesign a language is always negative: he restricts and excludes, scrubs and sterilizes, and ultimately impoverishes. The remarks of the nineteenth-century French historian and philologist Ernest Renan resound with the indignation of the genuine scholar.

> The grammarian who sets about reforming a language according to some preconceived system generally succeeds only in rendering it barren and colorless, sapping all its natural vigor and incidentally

leaving it no more "logical" than the most primitive dialect. . . .
He misses no opportunity of pointing out the inconsistencies and
want of logic that mar the language as the people have made it.
He sneers scornfully at the clumsiness of a merely traditional
system of speech, and presumes to correct each fault in the light
of grammatical "reason," blissfully unaware that the usages that
he wants to suppress are nearly always preferable to the ones that
he wants to substitute for them. The human intellect, when left to
its own devices, does not, cannot create anomalous patterns of
expression. The speech of children and illiterates is infinitely richer
than the dull jabbering of grammarians. In this as in so many
other things, the artificial productions of the self-appointed re-
former botch and spoil the work of nature, the only living and
true work. (Renan E: *De l'Origine du Langage* [1848], my
translation.)

The earliest English grammarians were too prone to judge their language by the yardstick of the classical languages. Persuaded that clarity
begins at Rome, they imposed Latin grammar on English and insisted
upon a strict etymological interpretation of words derived from Latin. A
large class of traditional English grammatical prohibitions are survivals
of Latin grammar.

The silliest crotchet of the older grammarians was their pathetic and
desperate determination to make the language remain static, as though
the dictionary were to be imposed by edict on the populace. In this we
see yet another result of the professional scholar's preoccupation with
dead, and hence fixed, languages. Prevented by the obstinacy or apathy
of the general public, if not by their own common sense, from amending
"inconsistencies" in the language, the grammarians struggled to keep
errors and variant usages from becoming general and so passing beyond
their bailiwick.

Phonetic and semantic changes are signs of life, health and growth in a
language. Even artificial languages begin to evolve (to the horror of their
inventors) as soon as large numbers of people learn them and put them
to use. The grammarian who wants to impose a decerebrate rigidity on
human speechways has yet to learn the basic truth that the variations as
well as the consistencies, the false analogies as well as the strict logic all
make up a language.

But we must not fall into the trap of excessive tolerance. The twentieth
century has seen two major revolutions in language study, structural
linguistics and transformational grammar. Each is a reaction against
what has gone before, and each studies language from a radically new
point of view. If regarded merely as revisions of traditional grammar,

they seem like elaborate but not very clever hoaxes. Revisions, however, they are not; they come up with different answers because they ask different questions. Their rules are like the laws of gravity or thermodynamics: they describe phenomena. They do not say, "Your sentence would be more intelligible if you made such and such a correction," but rather, "People understand such and such a construction to mean so and so."

This vigorous swing of the pendulum in the direction of a descriptive and almost speculative study of language has led to yet a further perversion of the grammarian's role and title. Though the point of view that regards a language as a law unto itself is a welcome respite from the strictures and oppressions of traditional grammar, it has seduced grammarians and educators alike into concentrating on "observed" language and refusing to recognize, much less endorse and teach, any kind of standard. From the notion that a language cannot go wrong it is but one step to the delusion that an individual user of the language cannot go wrong—even when no one can understand him.

THE PRINTED WORD

An especially pernicious tenet of this ultramodern school of grammar is that all standards peculiar to writing are to be rejected as artificial and accidental, a position with which everyone of intelligence and culture must violently disagree. No matter how much latitude we may tolerate in speech, even among professionals discussing abstract or complex subjects, weighty considerations dictate our setting up and following strict standards for formal writing. The ceaseless change that we recognize as so natural and necessary a feature of living speech much be curbed in some measure when we record our thoughts in print if they are to have widespread and enduring significance and usefulness. The printed word is a precision instrument, not a stick of dynamite or a sledgehammer.

It is self-evident that consistency belongs to the very essence of language. A word can represent and transmit an idea only as long as its significance is universally, or at least generally, accepted. "Words," wrote Hazlitt, "are like money, not the worse for being common. . . . It is the stamp of custom alone that gives them circulation and value."

A reader's ease and comfort depend on his absolute familiarity with each word that he sees. To spell a word in a variety of ways, to use it in unorthodox constructions, or to assemble needlessly intricate syntax confuses and distracts. Devotees of the frantic and thrill-packed sport known as speedreading claim that the practiced reader absorbs not merely syllables or words but whole phrases at one glance. In order to elicit a resonance of meaning each word and phrase must be not only instantly recognizable but perfectly unequivocal. Clearly this cannot be the case unless these words and phrases are used with perfect consistency.

Formal writing demands also a certain standard of elegance and decorum. The relation between writer and reader rests on mutual respect as well as a common ground of expression. Competence in standard English is a by-product of higher education (rarely, a direct result of elementary education). Readers of medical literature, as educated and cultivated professionals, expect anyone who claims their attention with a technical book or paper to use formal technical English exclusively and to use it correctly.

"Correctness" is an emotionally charged word, conjuring up notions of regimentation, legislation and restriction. We can identify not one but many standards of correctness in writing. When a horse breeder looks at a race horse, he considers its dimensions and proportions. A jockey is more interested in its surefootedness and docility. To a betting man these are of less importance than speed and stamina. Though all of these qualities are related, certain ones are singled out by the special viewpoint of each observer. Similarly, the logic of a piece of writing, its intelligibility and its conformity to general usage are broadly interrelated, but each may be separately applied as a measure of correctness.

Of these three standards the least important and least valid is logic. True logic in language is a will-o'-the-wisp, a mere figment of the grammarian's lack of imagination. No direct and necessary connection links word and idea. The only internal logic we can expect of language is a general conformity to certain basic patterns. That is what we mean when we say that language is analogical rather than logical.

Even when a locution fails to meet the test of analogy it may be tolerated if it is universally understood. Thus, though "The patient *could not seem* [seemed unable] to understand the directions," "He found *that his hat had become too small for him* [that his head had become too large for his hat]," and I couldn't *help* [avoid] hearing what you said" are neither logical nor analogical, we cannot on those grounds alone condemn them, since their wide currency gives them the stamp of usage and ensures their intelligibility.

Old grammar books railed vehemently against the illogical expression, "the best of all others." This phrase, almost never heard nowadays, was abolished not by the schoolmaster fighting under the banner of reason but simply by a shift of fashion. *Irregardless* and *unloosen* are just as illogical as "the best of all others," and just as old, but they survive and flourish because usage keeps them going.

Usage may be taken in either a broad or a narrow sense. In the broad sense it refers to a general consent among the speakers of a language as to the meaning of a word, phrase or construction. Quintilian had this sense in mind when he wrote, "Usage is the surest standard of correctness." It is upon this principle that the whole utility of language depends. That does not mean that change in language is undesirable, only that usage loses its title to determine correctness when it is not universal. In Osler's day it was the medicine that often proved nauseous; in ours it is the patient. Though at some future date everyone who says "nauseous" may mean "about to vomit," that is not the case now. Whether the word is used with its old or its new meaning, it will mislead some readers, at least at first glance. When usage is variable it ceases to be a valid standard of correctness and must yield the helm to intelligibility.

In a narrower sense usage may be taken to mean the speech habits peculiar to a region or socioeconomic group. In Memphis and New Orleans it is perfectly good English to speak of "feeling of a patient's abdomen." In Boston or Rochester, however, the preposition would be regarded as a superfluity and an abomination.

Social standards of usage are by far the most whimsical and troublesome. It has been said that there is no clear difference between a flower and a weed. Untrue: the difference is that if you cultivate weeds in your garden your neighbors will despise you, whereas if you cultivate flowers they probably will not. And that is the only difference. It does not reside in any intrinsic properties of the plants themselves but in the customary societal attitude toward them. I do not know how many millions of dollars Americans spend each year in cultivating ryegrass and roses, but I suspect we spend much more in exterminating crabgrass and dandelions.

Now, *isn't* and *anyhow* and *to whom* are flowers, whereas *ain't* and *nohow* and *to who* are weeds. The difference is not in the intrinsic properties of the words but in the attitude of "cultivated" society toward them. Nor do the cultivated alone harbor such attitudes, for linguistic chauvinism flourishes at every social stratum. Anyone who doubts this has probably never been present at an interview between an illiterate native American and a foreign medical graduate whose English was less than fluent.

Besides regional and social standards of usage, we must not forget that there is a sharp distinction between what is tolerated in speech and what is fit for formal writing. "The serum amylase came back elevated" is perfectly acceptable in conversation but it would be objectionably lax and colloquial in a technical paper.

Though the various standards based on usage may have a savor of snobbery and modishness about them, we must recognize them as matters of taste, and recall that to accommodate oneself to the tastes of others is the very essence of courtesy. We must also admit, though, that usage is a fickle judge. Its decisions are never final, and its laws are so changeable that no one can be perfectly abreast of them. Surely no dictionary can be perfectly accurate in recording them.

At the turn of the century the adjective *nearby,* as in "a nearby delicatessen," was regarded as a vulgarism, and school children were taught to avoid it like smallpox. Now it is acceptable in the most formal and sophisticated writing. What wrought this change was that those children paid less attention to what they heard in school than to what they heard everywhere else. *Nearby* illustrates not only shifting fashions in language but also the upward mobility of colloquialisms: yesterday's slang becomes tomorrow's formal usage.

"That there Dr. Fogbank is a real genius—he writes books as *nobody* can understand." Though the universal unintelligibility of Fogbank's works may mark him as a genius to the unsophisticated observer, to a more discerning critic it is a sign of his clumsiness and incompetence as a writer. Intelligibility is the final and most potent arbiter of correctness in writing. This point is so evident that it needs neither amplification nor defense. What cannot be understood is not language.

We are now in a position to survey the range covered by the grammarian's table of rules and precepts. At one end of the spectrum are principles of syntax which save the writer the trouble of judging whether a construction is understandable or not; at the other are the dictates of shifting and irrational fashions and archaic prejudices such as those against split infinitives and final prepositions.

Logic, usage and intelligibility overlap and interweave to such a degree that efforts to distinguish them in practice are usually futile. What violates one standard often violates the others as well. Examples of incorrect writing cited throughout this book are usually not accompanied by detailed analyses: the reader must expect to apply his own judgment in deciding why, and indeed whether, they are objectionable.

That there is more to good writing than grammatical correctness and the observance of social standards every intelligent reader will probably agree. Writing that is merely correct is not necessarily readable. A paper that contains no errors of spelling, grammar or punctuation, no regionalisms, vulgarisms or colloquialisms, may yet be dull, obscure, pompous, repetitious, rambling and self-contradictory. Techniques for achieving clarity, succinctness, coherence, vigor and variety in speech and writing are the province of the science of rhetoric. Whereas grammar concerns itself only with the forms of words and their "logical" arrangement in sentences, rhetoric takes a broader view, and seeks to make language both more appealing and more effective as a tool of communication. (I use *rhetoric* here in a technical sense. We have no concern with its other meaning, the black art of clothing falsehoods in the garb of truth and nonsense in the guise of logic.)

Because practical grammar and rhetoric are largely devoted to amending common errors, they have their negative and unattractive side. A code of civil law which dealt with the subjects of burglary, theft, robbery with violence, extortion, blackmail and embezzlement by simply stating the rule, "Everyone must be honest," would be of no conceivable use in protecting private property. Grammar and rhetoric are often most useful when they tell the writer what not to write and why.

It may be snobbery to claim that a physician who can write, "The question was as to where the stenosis was at" is not fit to tell his colleagues the answer with any degree of authority. But an entire paper couched in such vulgar, inept, tedious and distracting language would as surely fail to convey the author's thoughts with precision and clarity as it would repel most educated readers.

Modern medical writing, heavily edited though it is before it reaches print, offers abundant evidence of a need for a general improvement in clarity and readability. My object in writing this book has been to put together in succinct form some practical directions for the medical writer who aspires to a correct, concise and appealing style. On questions of usage and taste I have done my best to be descriptive rather than prescriptive, though of course a guide that refuses to adopt and sustain a position on shifting or variant usages can hardly exert any constructive influence. I have seen no need to be dogmatic or even didactic on matters of simple intelligibility, of which the reader can form his own judgments. Throughout the book my chief purpose has been not to teach a skill but to delineate an ideal and suggest means of attaining it.

REFERENCES

Barnett L: *The Treasure of Our Tongue*. New York, Alfred A Knopf, 1965.
Bloomfield MW, Newmark L: *A Linguistic Introduction to the History of English*. New York, Alfred A Knopf, 1963.
Bodmer F: *The Loom of Language*. New York, WW Norton & Co, 1944.
Dorsey JM: *Psychology of Language*. Detroit, Center for Health Education, 1971.
Jespersen O: *Language, Its Nature, Development and Origin*. New York, W W Norton & Co, 1964.
Matthews B: *Essays on English*. New York, Charles Scribner's Sons, 1921.
Potter S: *Modern Linguistics*. New York, WW Norton & Co, 1964.

2

The Technical Language of Medicine

Only a small part of the physician's working vocabulary consists of medical terminology properly so called, since most of the words he uses in speaking and writing about technical subjects are just ordinary English. In setting forth the principles of grammar and style later in this book I shall have much to say about the proper choice and arrangement of those ordinary English words. The present chapter, however, is limited to a discussion of technical terms.

The history of medical terminology parallels and mirrors the history of medicine itself. This relationship is particularly manifest when we survey the evolution of names for diseases. In the most primitive era, *jaundice* (or an equivalent term meaning "yellowness of the skin") was viewed as the name of a single disease. Later, when it was widely recognized that some jaundiced persons had pain whereas others did not, that some died whereas others recovered, *jaundice* became a generic term for a group of diseases, which were distinguished by descriptive markers or qualifiers such as *catarrhal* and *malignant*.

Still later, it became evident that jaundice was not so much a disease as a symptom or sign of excessive bile in the blood, a sign common to several otherwise unrelated disorders. The term then began to be qualified by pathogenetic markers such as *obstructive, hemolytic, toxic.* Meanwhile a new set of terms had come into being to designate the diseases and abnormal states known to cause jaundice: *cholelithiasis, hemolysis, hepatitis.* Though they marked a significant advance beyond the stage in which all such conditions were viewed as kinds of jaundice, these new terms were, like *jaundice* itself, largely descriptive.

Another cycle of advances began when causes of cholelithiasis, hemolysis and hepatitis were sorted out and identified, and a new set of pathogenetic markers—*cholesterol stones, Rh incompatibility, serum hepatitis*—came into use. As none of these causes is final in the metaphysical sense, neither the analytic process nor the revision of terminology can ever end. These activities may be retarded or arrested when further investigation seems unlikely to yield further gains in prevention or treatment, as in the case of many genetic abnormalities at the present time; or, on the other hand, when sufficient information has been gathered to permit effective control or prevention, as in the case of smallpox and polio. All the same, there is no such thing as a primary disease, unless one is so cynical as to regard human existence itself as fitting that description, as did the professional cynic Alexander Pope when he spoke of "this long disease, my life."

THE SOURCES OF MEDICAL TERMS

The derivations of the words and phrases that make up the formal technical terminology of medicine are so varied, and in some cases so tortuous and bizarre, that it may be of interest to trace some of them before we examine the standards governing the form and use of these terms. Such an inquiry is not without its practical side, since the medical writer, though not always the inventor of new terms, is their principal propagator.

Many of the most-used medical terms have been taken from lay English and date back much farther than modern scientific medicine. Some of these mean the same thing to the physician that they mean to the layman (*heart, measles, wound*) but others have acquired more restricted or even wholly different meanings (*block, tenderness, shock*). Though many English medical terms come of Anglo-Saxon stock, others entered our language from French during the Norman period (*pain, plague, bowel*). Besides English words of literal denotation, there are many which are used figuratively in medicine: *saddle block, hockey-stick incision, berry aneurysm, cherry angioma.*

Anyone who is even superficially acquainted with modern medical terminology knows that Latin and Greek play a dominant part in its composition. Some words have been taken over from the classical languages without much change in form—for example, *syncope* and *pharynx* from Greek, *axilla* and *delirium* from Latin. Others are compounds or derivatives built up in English from stems and affixes borrowed from Greek (*microaerophilic, pericardiectomy*) or Latin (*radiolucent, seroconversion*), from combinations of the two (*rectosigmoid, neurovascular*) or by mixture of classical material with English (*endartery, hemiblock*) or other languages, including medieval German (*antiscorbutic*) and Arabic (*alkalosis*).

Laymen sometimes accuse physicians of fabricating their abstruse jargon from dead languages so as to surround the lore of their craft with an awesome mystery. History, however, offers a different interpretation of the facts. For many centuries Latin served as the universal language of Western scholars, the official idiom of the republic of letters. Since it was the vehicle of most academic instruction in Europe, as well as the language of pre-Reformation Christianity and of jurisprudence, the terminologies of the arts, the sciences and the professions were built up in Latin rather than in vernacular languages. The fact that it was "dead," no longer the spoken tongue of any race on earth, only enhanced its value as a means of recording and diffusing information in fields of inquiry where definitions must remain fixed and denotations invariable.

Vesalius and Harvey, like Galileo and Newton, reported their scientific findings in a Latin that differed only in literary quality from the language of Cicero. In the sixteenth century Ambroise Paré outraged his colleagues by publishing the results of his surgical experiments in French instead of Latin, and as late as 1687 one Christian Thomasius was expelled from the University of Leipzig for presuming to lecture in German. The annual Harveian Oration was read in Latin before the Royal College of Physicians (London) until 1865.

A large part of medical Latin had its origin in pre-Christian times. In the first century A.D. Aulus Cornelius Celsus, probably not a physician himself, compiled a practical treatise on medicine in a Latin style remarkable for its purity and conciseness. The eight books of his *De Medicina* are a principal source of information about pre-Galenic medicine and its terminology. The modern reader is struck by the vast number of Greek terms which Celsus used. The Romans got along very nicely without doctors until they conquered Greece and took possession of the arts and sciences that pertained to the superior and more advanced Hellenic culture. Among these they found a fully developed science of medicine, complete with a technical jargon and a long-standing rivalry between "rationals" and "empirics."

Once introduced to the notion of a medical profession, the Romans displayed no great eagerness to enter such a profession themselves. For some centuries after the conquest of Greece, most medical practitioners in the Roman empire were Greek-speaking slaves or freemen, either from Greece itself or from Greek colonies in Egypt or the Near East. (In the second century Galen immigrated to Rome from Asia Minor.) Thus it came about that when Celsus wrote a Latin treatise on medicine he was compelled to use a technical nomenclature that was heavily saturated with Greek words. Though *asthma, erysipelas* and *zygoma* appear in *De Medicina* in Greek letters, other Greek terms (*arteria, carcinoma, thorax*) were already sufficiently naturalized in Celsus' day to be written in Roman letters and inflected like Latin words.

Despite the profusion of words borrowed at various periods from Greek, classical Latin had its own substantial lexicon of anatomic and pathologic terms, including *abdomen, femur, fistula* and *impetigo.* The language of the early medieval anatomists was ordinary lay Latin. Thus, *pollex = thumb, brachium = arm* and *vesica urinaria = urinary bladder* were intelligible to anyone who knew Latin, not just to physicians and anatomists. When the anatomist needed a name for a newly discovered structure, he took a classical or later Latin word and applied it metaphorically.

From the wardrobe of the Romans of the Augustan era, for example, he borrowed *tunica* (a light garment for indoor wear), *zona = belt or girdle, fascia = band, bursa = purse* and *fibula = brooch, safety pin.* In this figurative labeling of parts of the body with common words the anatomists of the Middle Ages were only following the lead of their classical predecessors. Already in Galen's time the practice of naming a part after something which it resembled in shape was so prevalent that a few structures that seemed unlike anything else had to be left "innominate," that is, nameless. Pathologic nomenclature also included metaphors from earliest times: Hippocrates wrote of *lagophthalmos = hare's eye,* Celsus of *kynanche = a dog's choke-halter* (now corrupted to *quinsy*), Galen of *pterygion = little wing.*

Once a metaphor gets started it is apt to sprout new meanings with the passing centuries. Latin *cratera* (adapted from Greek *krater*) meant a serving bowl or a cup; by transference, a bowl-shaped depression in the earth (cf. *pot-hole*), then the hollow of a volcano. The radiologist's term *ulcer crater* extends the metaphor yet further.

Some Latin words have been pressed into service so many times over that their aptness has worn thin and their utility has waned proportionately. To the ancient Romans a *sinus* was a curve or bend. In Augustan days the word referred to a fold customarily placed in the upper part of the toga, allowing freedom to the right arm and also serving as a large pocket. In modern anatomy the extension of sinus includes mucosa-lined cavities adjacent to the nasal space, venous pools in the cerebral circulation, bulbous dilatations in the carotid arteries, widenings at the root of the aorta from which the coronary arteries arise, potential spaces between the folds of the pericardium, a chamber of the fetal heart as well as its permanent representative adjacent to the right atrium, fusiform bulges of the lactiferous ducts, pleural spaces between the lower ribs and the diaphragm, pear-shaped recesses adjacent to the larynx, a collecting gutter for the prostatic ducts, a fold between the body of the epididymis and the testis, the embryonic precursor of the lower urinary tract, and the canal of communication between the aqueous humor and the scleral veins.

Medical Latin does not, of course, consist entirely of figures of speech. Many terms are straightforward descriptive adjectives (*rotundum, ellipticus, rubrum, niger*). A number of these act as nouns, since their original companion nouns are customarily dropped: [*arteria*] *trachea = rough artery* (Greek); *dura* [*mater*] = *tough membrane;* [*nervus*] *vagus* = *wandering nerve;* [*membrana*] *mucosa;* [*musculus*] *rectus* = *straight muscle.* Each of these terms preserves the gender of the dropped noun. (*Calcaneus,* for *os calcaneum,* is an inexplicable modern corruption.) In the case of [*intestinum*] *rectum* = *straight gut* the "noun" is itself a neuter adjective (*intestinum* = *internal*).

Medical Latin has been steadily augmented down through the centuries, but at an ever-slackening rate. The ancient Romans did not use stirrups, but by the time that the stirrup-shaped bone of the middle ear needed a name, medieval Latin had one for it: *stapes,* perhaps from *stare* = *to stand* and *pes* = *foot.* Musculus sartorius, the tailor's muscle, had to wait for its name until tailors came into being and used this muscle to assume their customary crosslegged working position. The Augustans had no tailors and no such word as *sartorius. Rubella* and *rubeola* (both from *rubrum* = *red*) and *morbilli* (originally *morbillus* = *little disease*) date from the early modern era.

Neo-Latin is being coined even in our own day (*foetor hepaticus, status anginosus*), sometimes with a freedom that pains the classicist. The nomenclature of skin diseases includes many abstruse Latin terms, primarily descriptive, which in some cases have proliferated to an unreasonable extent. Thus, papular urticaria may also be called lichen urticatus, strophulus infantum, strophulus pruriginosus or prurigo simplex acuta. *Purpura hypergammaglobulinemica,* an attempt at etiologic naming, is unwieldy with its eight-morpheme, ten-syllable adjective.

Linnaean taxonomy (which to the physician denotes almost exclusively the classification of pathogenic microorganisms) also continues to fabricate names which are Latin in form, though the stems are more often Greek. For example, the Loch Ness monster has lately been dubbed *Nessiteras rhombopteryx.* (See Naming the Loch Ness monster (editorial). *Nature* (London) 258:466-468, 1975.) Since viruses are not living organisms they have hitherto been excluded from the Linnaean system, as their chaotic and anamalous nomenclature plainly shows.

Modern medicine, as though fearful of exhausting the lexical resources of the classical languages, avidly snatches up words from other living languages (*espundia, kuru, spinnbarkeit*). Borrowing words from languages other than Latin and Greek is by no means a purely modern practice, however. Many such medical borrowings date from the Middle Ages: *bezoar* from Persian, *saphena* from Arabic, *malaria* from Italian.

The classical traditions that dominated Western culture from the Renaissance to the early part of the present century saturated the imaginations of scholars with figures and fancies drawn from Greek and Roman mythology. Many terms in modern medicine derive their significance from these myths: *Minerva jacket, Venus' girdle, Delphian nodes.*

While continuing the practice in a modest way, twentieth-century medicine has not hesitated to draw terms from more modern literature (*Munchausen syndrome, Pickwickian syndrome*). Most proper names in medicine, however, are eponymic (*addisonian, bartholinitis, Castellani's paint, Devic's disease, Ewing's sarcoma*), with geographic terms (*Mediterranean anemia, Hong Kong influenza*) far behind in second place.

BRAVE NEW WORDS

The borrowing of words from other languages and the extension of common words to special meanings do not suffice to meet the needs of a constantly expanding discipline. By far the most fruitful source of terms added to the medical lexicon in the past century has been the process of coinage or neoterism. Very few neoterisms are brand new, virtually all being composed of morphemes (usually from the classical languages) which are already endowed with meaning.

The practice of combining two or more words (free morphemes) in a single lexical unit such as *afterbirth, fingernail* and *seasick* is found in nearly all languages, and was already well developed in Greek by Homer's time. Many of the stock epithets for characters in the *Iliad* and the *Odyssey* are composite nouns or adjectives: *Zeus nephelegereta* = *the cloud gatherer, Athene glaukopsis* = *the grey-eyed*. The name of Oedipus, the king of ancient Thebes whose tragic fate has fired the imaginations of so many dramatists and psychiatrists, is another compound (*oidipous* = *swollen foot*).

Sclerocardia, which every physician can translate on sight as "hardness of heart," appears in the Septuagint version of the Old Testament (before 100 B.C.). This term illustrates two features of word coinage that have survived to the present day: the use of an extraneous vowel (in this case *o*) to link two stems, and the addition of an affix, or bound morpheme (here, the suffix *-ia,* meaning *a condition or state*).

The formation of a compound may be viewed as the terminal stage in a process of compression through which a complex idea comes to be represented by a single word. In the first stage the idea is, or could be, expressed by a phrase containing prepositions or conjunctions or both: "lowering of the sugar in the blood," "inflammation of the joint between sacrum and ilium," "cutting into the membrane between the cricoid and thyroid cartilages." In successive stages of condensation the phrase loses its prepositions ("blood sugar lowering"), perhaps being partly translated into technical terms of classical origin ("sacroiliac arthritis"), and is finally concentrated into a single word: *hypoglycemia, sacroiliitis, cricothyrotomy.* Often yet a further stage occurs, in which the word originally formed is shortened by syncopation of unwanted syllables. Thus, *hemo-*

globin and *aryepiglottic* first saw the light of day as *haematinoglobulin* and *arytaenoepiglottidean*. An entire stem sometimes vanishes from a compound in the process of abridgment, as in *thrombopenia* from *thrombocytopenia*.

There is practically no limit to the variety of patterns possible in composition and affixation. We can join two nouns to form a third: *pyosalpinx, pneumothorax*. We can make a new adjective from two others: *cardiovascular, ileojejunal*. We can attach an adjective permanently to a noun: *erythrocyte, megacolon*. With a prefix we can qualify a noun (*hypophysis, exophthalmos*) or imbed in it a prepositional phrase (*hypothalamus, epiglottis*). With a suffix we can change the species of a noun (*ptyalism, psychosis*) or convert it into an adjective (*neuronal*), a verb (*chelate*), even an adverb or preposition (*caudad*).

No longer is there much reluctance, as there once was, to mix Latin and Greek material together. Nearly all modern medical suffixes (*-itis, -osis, -ectomy, -otomy, -oma, -emia, -algia, -odynia*) are Greek. Because of the old prejudice against combining Greek and Latin lexical material, many Greek stems were drawn into the medical language for coupling with these suffixes, even though the anatomic nomenclature already contained Latin words for the parts in question. Hence such unnecessary duplications as *dermal-cutaneous, xiphoid-ensiform* and *scaphoid-navicular*. (See Dirckx JH: Hybrid words in medical terminology. *JAMA,* in press.)

The insatiable thirst of some writers for a succinct way to express each concept (which, curiously enough, often coexists with an unbridled passion for circumlocution and verbosity) has led to a coalescence of stems and affixes in a dense morphemic matrix without rule or principle. Though it may be unreasonable to expect perfect logic or perfect consistency in a naturally evolving language, it is not only reasonable but necessary that an artificial system of nomenclature adhere rigidly to established forms and patterns.

There could be no better model of this regularity than chemical terminology, whose serried ranks of *-ic* and *-ous*, *-ate* and *-ite*, *-ane, -ene* and *-one,* infinitely more orderly and predictable than the paradigms of any natural language, are for that very reason instantly and universally understood. By comparison, the formal terminology of medicine is alphabet soup. The classical rhetoricians directed that three qualities should distinguish every new word: necessity, analogy and euphony. Let us see in what ways medical coinages are most conspicuously delinquent.

Necessity: *A new word should supply a deficiency.* Surely this rule, at least, needs no defense. The number of terms which the modern physician must carry in his head is so huge that only the most compelling of reasons can justify further additions to it. The baseless conviction that everything in medicine must have its own one-word name is not such a reason, and neither is the itch to add one's personal contribution to the already bursting medical lexicon. When a phrase of two or even three familiar words identifies something clearly, precisely and distinctively, it is idle and pernicious to fabricate a new word for it.

Besides new compounds, medical language is prolific of irregular derivatives and corruptions that compete with and sometimes drive out older and more legitimate terms. When we can say with perfect correctness that veins become *varicose,* why should we tolerate the slang mutation *varicosed?* Why say that a patient was found *cyanosed* when we have so much more suitable a term in *cyanotic? To obtund* is to dull or blunt. Though the intellect or the senses may be obtunded, it is cant to say, "The patient was obtunded." More to our present purpose, *obtundation* is a modern, anomalous and rather ugly variant of the established and correct *obtusion. To replete* has been fashioned from *repletion,* apparently on the analogy of *deplete.* The correct English word is *replenish.* The *Oxford English Dictionary* lists *to replete* as an obsolete verb; there seems to be no reason to resurrect it. *Anovulatory,* though a Greek-Latin hybrid, seems plain and proper enough, but its offshoot *anovulation* is a painfully irregular substitute for *nonovulation.* Immunosuppression and anticoagulation may have been inevitable, but must we say that patients are *immunosuppressed* and *anticoagulated?*

Analogy: *A new term should be formed by analogy with existing terms.* It is bad enough to add a new word to the dictionary whenever a new technique, instrument, pathologic change or species of lunacy must be reported. It is worse to coin a term whose general meaning is not readily apparent to the professional reader, and worse yet to concoct one that seduces the reader or hearer into a misinterpretation through false analogy with older words. The expected conformity to existing terms is threefold:

1. *A new word should contain stems and affixes already current in medical terminology.* So vast a swarm of Greek and Latin stems and affixes are already in service that there could not conceivably be a need to call in many more. The practice of ferreting out some hitherto-unused word from a Latin dictionary or a Greek lexicon as raw material for a novel and unique coinage should be strongly discouraged. A classical stem which has no derivatives in current medical terminology is not more apt or meaningful than a pure invention.

2. *Stems and affixes should be used with standard or established meanings.* The goal of perfect consistency does not necessarily demand that each stem preserve its classical sense. The extensive role of metaphor in medical nomenclature would alone render that impossible. All the

same, an appeal to parent words is sometimes needed to resolve sibling rivalry among their descendants.

Some modern terms are exactly like obsolete ones with entirely different meanings. *Anthracosis* once meant a boil, and *fibrillation* was formerly a morphologic feature, not a malfunction. Though *arachnoid* now means *like a cobweb,* in classical writings it meant *like a spider.* Even *urinate* formerly meant something quite different: *to dive.* (See Oleson JP: A possible physiological basis for the term *urinator,* "diver." *Am J Philol* 97:22-29, 1976.)

Whether or not a stem is used in its classical sense, it should preserve the same sense in all new coinages. As medical terminology grows in bulk, its coherence and internal associations become looser. Stems acquire increasingly divergent meanings, so that the consistency that is essential for intelligibility is gradually lost. As in natural language, each morpheme comes to have an approximate and general significance as new connotations are added to its denotation.

Moreover, the denotation itself may be lost. The literal meaning of *parenteral,* from *para = beside* and *enteron = bowel,* is "(administered by a route) other than the digestive system." The word was apparently not coined until after the development of the hollow needle, and there is evidence to show that from the first it has referred exclusively to injections. The denotation of *parenteral* is thus preserved in the statement, "Metronidazole is not available in parenteral form." (Though it is marketed in vaginal inserts as well as oral tablets, metronidazole is not at this writing available in injectable form.) But what of the denotation of the morphemes that make up *parenteral?* As has lately been observed, *nonparenteral* is an equivocal and unsatisfactory way of saying *other than injectable.* (See Greenbaum DS: Where is "nonparenteral"? *NEJM* 291: 51, 1974 and Makris CH: "Nonparenteral" means "enteric." *JAMA* 234:1223, 1975.)

The lack of any absolute scheme or rule according to which the elements of a compound coinage are to be put together sometimes renders a polymorphemic compound ambiguous or even unintelligible. As in the case of *nonparenteral,* a pileup of prefixes is particularly apt to confuse: *biodegradable, nonextrapyramidal, polyunsaturate, undiversion.* The variation between *amyotrophic* and *myasthenic* in the relative positions of *a = without* and *my(o)- = muscle* is purely arbitrary.

Even when coinage proceeds along fairly narrow and disciplined lines, it often happens that a stem or affix acquires several vaguely related meanings. The reader who is obliged to guess may thus find himself in the right church but the wrong pew. The stem *phag-,* from the Greek verb meaning *to eat,* is stretched metaphorically in various directions by *macro-*

phage (a tissue cell that engulfs things), *bacteriophage* (a virus that invades bacteria) and *vitreophage* (an instrument that sucks out the vitreous humor). *Path-* may refer to either disease or treatment, and *gen-* to either cause or result. (See Gode A: Just words. *JAMA* 182:608, 1962 and 190: 999, 1964; Buck RW: Iatral, not iatrogenic. *NEJM* 294:1298, 1976.) Fabricators of new terms should take pains to avoid not only stems of variable connotation but also those which represent two or more parent words (*osm-, onc-, io[n]-*).

Affixes, too, are apt to be employed inconsistently. In *preoperative* and *prepuberal* the prefix acts as a preposition meaning *before,* but in *prefrontal* and *pretibial* as a preposition meaning *in front of.* In *prerenal* (azotemia) and *prehepatic* (jaundice) the notions of priority and anteriority are subtly intertwined. The prefix completely loses its prepositional character in *pre-existing* and *preformed,* serving instead as an adverb meaning earlier. In *prediabetes* and *preleukemia* it is an adjective meaning latent or impending, while in *pre-excitation* it means early or premature.

The composite suffix *-uria* denotes an abnormality of the urine in *hematuria, chyluria* and *pyuria,* but refers to the act of voiding in *nocturia, dysuria* and *anuria.* Even suffixes in common use in the lay language are often pressed into variant and anomalous roles. The Latin participle and supine ending *-atus* (*-atum*) is a prolific source of derivative words in medical English (*distillate, filtrate*), including many with Greek (*hydrolysate*) or even Anglo-Saxon (*leachate*) stems. Though these four examples all function as participles, other words formed with *-ate* are verbs, some of them back-formations (*chelate*), others simple coinages (*extubate*), and still others chemical or pharmaceutical inventions (*sulfate, morrhuate, clofibrate*).

Though some might object to the irregularity of a word like *anorexiant,* it at least preserves the meaning of the present (active) participle ending *-ant. Receptant,* however, recently proposed for any substance "received" by a receptor, has been justly condemned on the grounds that it implies an active rather than a passive receiving. (Vaisrub S: Terminological logic. *JAMA* 237:268, 1977.) We are reminded of the wild abandon with which officialese forms adjectives with *-able: grievable issue,* one subject to official grievance procedure; *removable offense,* one punishable by removal of the offender from employment. These are after all no worse than *fashionable, knowledgeable, sensible* and *serviceable.*

3. *Combining forms of classical stems should follow established patterns.* Though the form in which a Greek or Latin stem appears in modern terminology may vary greatly from classical models of correctness, it should match other modern forms of the stem.

The combining form of a classical word generally consists of the stem and a linking vowel. In scientific terms, combining forms are often shorter than in classical words. From an early date it has been a common practice to lop the last syllable from a stem: *tenosynovitis* for *tenonto-synovitis, hemochromatosis* for *hematochromatosis, plasmapheresis* for *plasmatapheresis.* The suffix *-oid* is usually dropped out of combining forms: *hyoid* → *hyoglossus, thyroid* → *thyrothymic.* Similarly, chemical suffixes are apt to seem expendable: *hypocholesteremia, sulfhemoglobin.* In *carotidynia* it is part of the second component (*odyne*) that has vanished. A compound containing a duplicated syllable may be telescoped by haplology: *Pulmotor, surfactant, volumetric, cephalgia* (the latter not yet quite respectable).

Nowadays a combining form is particularly apt to be built up from something other than a stem, most often either an unaltered nominative (*mucormycosis, apexcardiogram, sinusoid*) or an anomalous stem that lacks a final consonant (*ir* [*id*] *itis, orchi* [*d*] *opexy*) or preserves the final consonant of the nominative (*psoriasiform* for *psoriatiform*). *Metastatic* and *synthetase* contain the correct verb stems despite the unwholesome example of *metastasize* and *synthesize. Syphilidean* would be more conventional than *syphilitic, anorectic* than *anorexic, amniac* than *amniotic.* Sometimes a fragment is arbitrarily split from a word to serve as a combining form, as in *parathormone* and *prostaglandin.*

Modern terms vary widely in their choice of a linking vowel. Though combining forms of Latin stems were once regularly made with a linking *i* (*talipes, torticollis*), the *o* that has always been typical of Greek now prevails even with Latin stems. The *i*, however, has fused with certain suffixes of Latin origin: it almost always precedes *-cidal, -cide, -form* and *-fy* (*amebicidal, acneiform, esterify*), though with *-genic* it is variable: *tumori-genic, psychogenic,* even *asthmagenic* and *mutagenic.* The blatantly irregular *virucidal* has apparently come to stay. The lack of uniformity in linking vowels is evident in the series *reovirus, orbivirus, rotavirus* and *herpesvirus.* In the last example there is neither stem nor linking vowel. Though this is the usual pattern in English (*gallstone, frostbite*), classical material has traditionally been put together with classical cement.

Euphony: *A new word should be pleasing to the ear and in keeping with good taste.* Though euphony is not the most important consideration, it ought not to be neglected entirely. The coiner of a new term would probably be pardoned by all but the most fanatical purists for taking liberties with the shape of a stem in order to achieve a more pleasing sound, or even just a simpler one. This principle may justify the majority of delinquencies and aberrations recorded in the preceding section.

Some modern medical terms, however, offend good taste and common sense. The advertiser has nearly exhausted the possibilities of *mini-* and *maxi-, -matic* and *-tron,* and the medical profession would be well advised to leave these faddish morphemes alone. Even *de-* and *re-* have been somewhat overworked (*deconditioning, reuptake*). The past fifteen years have witnessed *The Pill's* grim progress from the tabloids through the slick newsmagazines to the medical literature. Though *sick cell syndrome* and *sick sinus syndrome* may be catchy, they lack the explicitness and sobriety that should distinguish the formal terminology of a scientific discipline. *Nonrheumatoid rheumatoid nodules* and *pseudopseudohypoparathyroidism* are likewise unduly whimsical and inexact.

MEDICAL LATIN

Latin became the language of anatomy, pathology and pharmacy because, though not a living tongue, it was understood everywhere. It has now died a second death: having dropped out of the high-school curriculum as well as the deliberations and promulgations of Church and State, it is understood as a language almost nowhere. To the nineteenth century medical student the meanings of *filum terminale* and *extensor digiti quinti proprius* were instantly apparent. If, as was more than likely, he had had a year or two of Greek, he also understood *tachycardia* and *phlebolith* on sight. Pharmaceutical abbreviations made perfect sense to him once he knew which Latin words they stood for. He was above such blunders, commonplace nowadays, as *condyloma lata, these papilla,* and *that strata.*

The medical Latin of today, with its incorrect plurals, dropped genitives, false concords and misplaced accents, is not Latin at all but a mangled "pidgin" dialect. The modern physician's knowledge of classical languages is limited to a nodding acquaintance with a vast hoard of isolated words and affixes, which are so constantly misinterpreted and misused that their meanings are in a perpetual state of transition and flux. The Latin of medicine is literally a language gone to seed.

Scabies means *the itch;* it is not plural and it certainly does not refer to mites, whose existence Horace and Celsus probably never suspected. In modern medical parlance, however, itch mites are frequently designated *scabies,* and drugs to kill them are called *scabicides.* To change the subject only slightly, though *pediculus = little foot* aptly names the various species of head and body louse, it is inaccurate to extend pediculosis to include infestation with crab lice. "Pediculosis due to *Phthirus pubis*" is as flagrant a contradiction in terms as "Tularemia due to *Corynebacterium diphtheriae.*"

It would be idle pedantry to object to modern pronunciations of classical words as "corruptions." English naturally tends to move the accent of a word forward (*VERTigo, TINNitus*) and to impose its own patterns of pronunciation on imported words, rhyming *rabies* with *babies* and *fomites* with *fleabites.* In writing for publication, however, one is expected to spell

Latin and latinized Greek terms in strict accord with modern practice, and to preserve the inflectional endings which carry so great a part of the meaning in an inflected language. Mutilated classical terms and phrases mar and cheapen a piece of writing. If approximate rather than exact grammar and spelling are not tolerated in English, why should they be tolerated in Latin, where meaning is so much more intimately linked to form?

The plurals of classical words have given trouble from time immemorial, and many unorthodox forms have attained legitimacy through long use. Though many Greek and Latin words can be pluralized in the English manner by the addition of -s or -es, a significant number are still expected to form their plurals according to classical rules. When current usage allows a choice, it is clearly preferable to use -s or -es (*scleras, ictuses*) rather than to commit a solecism (*sclerata, icti*) through ignorance of Latin.

Words ending in -a are perhaps the most fertile sources of confusion. Some of these that are singular are frequently taken to be plural (*ameba, stria, pleura*), and some that are plural are treated as singulars (*milia, media, strata*), often being made into double plurals (*septae, prodromata*). Some singulars ending in -a form their plurals in one way (*amebae*) and some in another (*zygomata*). The plurals of nouns ending in -us may be formed with -i (*radii*) or -a (*corpora*), or they may be unchanged from the singular (*meatus*). When the simple -s plural of a word is clearly not acceptable, a writer should verify the correct classical plural in a dictionary. By far the most useful and authoritative source of information on such points is *Stedman's Medical Dictionary* (see References at the end of this chapter).

Latin phrases containing prepositions (*aditus ad antrum, erythema ab igne, fistula in ano, amblyopia ex abusu*) are best avoided, but when used they must be spelled correctly. The grammatical issues that most often confound and embarrass the modern medical writer concern genitives and noun-adjective concords.

The genitive of a noun is its possessive form (the *patient's* shoes, The Library *of Congress*), though it may be used to show many other relations. The English genitive will be discussed in Chapter 4 with the grammar of the English noun; here we are concerned with the Latin genitive. Examples from both languages below illustrate common uses of the genitive besides showing simple possession.

PARTS, PROPERTIES, QUALITIES: the patient's shoulder, the odor of ripe fruit, the climate of Switzerland, toxemia of pregnancy

tendo Achillis, cervix uteri, ala nasi, muscularis mucosae

POSITION OR CONTIGUITY: the round ligament of the liver, carcinoma of the stomach

appendix testis, tinea cruris, pseudotumor cerebri

ORIGIN OR ESSENCE: oil of cloves, tincture of iodine

spiritus frumenti, liquor carbonis detergens

AGENCY OR CAUSE: the virus of mumps, the metabolic error of gout

Salmonella typhi, Mycoplasma pneumoniae

AUTHORSHIP OR DISCOVERY: Osler's works, Osler's nodes, the valves of Houston, Ringer's lactate

torcular Herophili, *Trypanosoma cruzi*

SUBJECTIVE GENITIVE: extravasation of urine, palpitations of the heart

pruritus ani, roseola infantum, concretio cordis

OBJECTIVE GENITIVE: avulsion of the nail, exploration of the abdomen

abruptio placentae, tensor tympani

The usual error involving the Latin genitive is an incorrect substitution of a nominative, the so-called missed genitive: *chondromalacia patella* for *patellae, abruptio placenta* for *placentae, muscularis mucosa* for *mucosae, H. influenza* for *influenzae, Coryne. acne* for *acnes*. These errors apparently arise from false analogy with a few phrases in which the genitive happens to be the same as the nominative (*appendix textis, corpus cavernosum penis*) or perhaps with phrases that contain no genitive at all (*placenta praevia*).

False concord occurs when a Latin adjective does not agree with its noun in gender, number and case. Here again the error usually results from a mistaken analogy. In many phrases the endings of noun and adjective are identical: *polycythemia vera; ligamentum flavum; pulsus rarus, parvus et tardus*. The principle on which such concords are based is not, however, one of rhyme but of inflectional pattern. Hence *lymphedema tarda, labium majorum* and *pectus excavatus* are wrong, the correct adjectives being *tardum, majus* and *excavatum*. On questions of concord, as of plurals, *Stedman's Medical Dictionary* is an invaluable guide for the perplexed.

There is, incidentally, no need to carry this matter of concord to extremes by enforcing it on phrases made up of anglicized Latin words.

Though *anterior septum, optimum status* and *minimum data* are abominable Latin, they are perfectly good English. My remarks on the grammar of medical Latin in this section apply strictly to terms and phrases already in use. The soundest advice to the physician who proposes to coin a new Latin phrase can be summed up in a single word: Don't.

EPONYMS

Strictly speaking an eponym is a person after whom something is named: George Washington is the eponym of the nation's capital, not the reverse. But in modern medical parlance, an eponym is usually taken to mean a term that contains or is derived from the name of a person: *Peyer's patches, addisonian, chagoma.* The person so commemorated is not necessarily the inventor or discoverer of the thing named. *Musset's sign* is named after the French author who had it, not the physician who first described it. The *spigelian lobe* of the liver was described by Adriaan van den Spieghel but the *spigelian hernia* was not, having been named after him because he first wrote about the linea semilunaris, in which it occurs.

Besides stirring up bitter disputes over priority of discovery, proper names in technical terminology create many vexing puzzles as to pronunciation and spelling. Because they are semantically inert they are difficult to learn. An eponym may refer to more than one thing (*Paget's disease*), and two or more eponyms may refer to the same thing (*Little's area, Kiesselbach's area*). Names with prepositions or conjunctions (*von Gierke, Ramón y Cajal*) present problems in alphabetization, as do double names (*Austin Flint, Ramsay Hunt, Tay-Sachs, Parkes-Weber*). (See Litt JZ: "Ramsay Hunt, Ramsay-Hunt or Hunt's Syndrome?" *JAMA* 236:345 - 346, 1976.) For obscure reasons the Christian names of Austin Flint, Graham Steell and Dorothy Reed, to mention a few, almost invariably accompany their surnames. The British practice of calling a man by his middle and last names (*Conan Doyle, Bernard Shaw*) adds to the confusion. James Ramsay Hunt and Henry Bence Jones belong with the *H*'s and the *J*'s respectively. A hyphen does not necessarily show that a double name refers to two persons: *Paul-Bunnell* are two persons, *Parkes-Weber* is one. Both terms belong with the *P*'s.

A peculiar innovation in styling lately adopted by some journals is the prohibition of the *'s* genitive in eponymic terms. Thus, *Hodgkin disease, Burow solution* and *Bell palsy* are written instead of the expected and long-established *Hodgkin's, Burow's* and *Bell's,* on the somewhat tenuous grounds that such terms do not show possession. (See Archer J: Epitomes. *JAMA* 234:152, 1975.) As demonstrated in the preceding section, the genitive denotes many relationships other than possession, conspicuous among these being discovery and authorship. We might say *Pike Peak* and *Halley comet* but we do not because the genitive form seems more natural. To insist upon a universal abolition of the *'s* genitive from eponyms is to make a fetish of uniformity by suppressing a natural feature of language.

Since genitives will of necessity continue to appear in taxonomic terms (*Rickettsia prowazekii, Wucheraria bancrofti*) and in ordinary discourse ("Dr. Molton's earlier technique," "Schaudinn's identification of the causative organism"), and since eliminating genitives formed with *of* (*island of Reil, pouch of Douglas*) would demand too drastic a reshaping of such terms, the stylistic uniformity is after all only illusory. The feeble and irrelevant argument that the person after whom a disease is named did not have that disease himself is not even universally true: Pott did have a Pott's fracture, and Carrión not only contracted Carrión's disease but died of it. No sooner had full genitives been restored to the AMA publications after an absence of about two years than they disappeared from *Postgraduate Medicine.* (See Howard RB: One man meat. *Postgrad Med* 62:22, July 1977.)

With or without apostrophes, proper names ending in *s* often give trouble, appearing in such mutilated versions as *Coomb's test* and *Homan sign.* In each of the following names the final *s* is integral, not a sign of the genitive: Adams, Archimedes, Chagas, Colles, Coombs, Danlos, Ehlers, Graves, Homans, Meigs, Perthes, Simmonds, Stokes, Weeks.

REFERENCES

Cole F: *The Doctor's Shorthand.* Philadelphia, W B Saunders Co, 1970.
Dirckx JH: *The Language of Medicine.* New York, Harper & Row, 1976.
Hyde LS (ed): *A Discursive Dictionary of Health Care.* Washington, DC, US Government Printing Office, 1976.
Leider M, Rosenblum M: *A Dictionary of Dermatological Words, Terms, and Phrases,* rev ed. West Haven, Conn, Dome Laboratories, 1976.
Stedman's Medical Dictionary, ed 23. Baltimore, Williams & Wilkins, 1976.

II

Sentences and Paragraphs:
The Physiology of Language

3

Medical Writing

WRITER AND EDITOR

The typical physician puts millions of words on paper during his professional career. Medical records, correspondence and official forms of diverse origins claim his attention during part of every working day and often nibble away at his leisure time as well. His handwriting deteriorates into an arcane hieroglyphic that is the despair of nurses and secretaries and an unfailing source of inspiration to amateur and professional comedians.

But penmanship is not our concern, and neither is most of what doctors write. The physician's technical writing can be divided into four broad classes, which I list here in order of increasing importance, elaborateness and formality.

1. Entries made in patients' records, impromptu and generally in longhand. Admitting and progress notes are perhaps the chief representatives of this class, but histories and physicals, operative reports and discharge summaries belong here too even though they are more often dictated than written. This material is historical and descriptive, refers to a specific patient, and is addressed to no one. It may never be read.

2. Record entries, correspondence, and other documents addressed to another physician, a nurse, pharmacist, physical therapist, laboratory technician or other health professional, perhaps even an attorney or an insurance company, providing information about a patient or requesting a service for him. This class includes orders in inpatient charts, prescriptions, consultation reports, case summaries and abstracts.

3. Writing addressed to a small group for teaching or administrative purposes: case protocols for clinicopathologic conferences, grand rounds

or seminars, summaries, charts, bibliographies and lecture "handouts." Even when the material refers to a single patient, the benefit of that patient (who may be dead) is not of primary concern in the writing.

4. Writing intended for publication, that is, wide dissemination in print: scientific papers and clinical reports in the medical literature, books or book chapters. This is what is principally meant by "medical writing," though that term properly includes technical exposition on any subject related to medical science, such as biochemistry, pharmacologic studies in animals, sanitation and psychoanalysis. In this book "medical writing" does not refer to popularized treatments of medical topics addressed to a lay audience, advertising copy, or articles written in "throwaway" magazine style.

Though my exclusive concern will be medical writing that is destined to appear in print, a physician who devotes some effort to the cultivation of a clear and pleasing style of formal writing will almost certainly improve his impromptu writing and dictating habits as well. Strengthening his grasp and command of language will also enhance the orderliness and validity of his thinking. (See Woodford FP: Sounder thinking through clearer writing. *Science* 156:743-745, 1967.)

It would be hard to overstate the role which technical exposition has played in the development and perfection of the science of medicine. Who today would know of Hippocrates or Galen, Averroes or Maimonides, Harvey or Heberden, much less revere them as prophets and pioneers, if they had not committed their observations to writing? How could the modern practitioner keep abreast of advances in medical science without access to the voluminous periodical literature of medicine? For a perceptive and stimulating account of the process by which scientific knowledge is gradually assembled from the contributions of many individual workers, see Ziman JM: Information, communication, knowledge. *Nature* (London) 224:318-324, 1969. See also Soffer A: Journals, clinicians and medical trends. *JAMA* 237:1966, 1977.

Why should a physician writing for publication take the trouble to polish his writing and make it clear, succinct and vigorous? As Hussey has lately pointed out, the constant stream of articles in the medical literature urging physicians to write better has had no obvious result. He suggests that because physicians are not often financially rewarded by their writing, they are not often motivated to write well. (Hussey HH: Medical writing: faults. *JAMA* 235:2327-2328, 1976.)

It is surely unnecessary to defend accuracy and clarity as important qualities in formal technical communication. The damage done by careless writing goes far beyond mere semantic and syntactic inefficiency. Language, as I remarked in an earlier chapter, is behavior: it reveals much about its user. Sloppy language repels and disgusts as surely as uncouth table manners or a predilection for dishabille and dirt. A reader can be forgiven for concluding that a writer who will not submit himself to the discipline of exact expression is probably deficient also in the intellectual self-discipline that befits a scientist and scholar.

A writer who cannot be troubled to keep his words and sentences in order is inevitably suspected of carelessness with facts and principles. Though the absentminded professor, that venerable stock-character of American folklore, no doubt has his counterparts in the real world, haphazard and slovenly habits of mind are scarcely compatible with the capacity to impart information in a clear and orderly manner. When medical writing comes under the scrutiny of members of other professions and of the learned disciplines—belles-lettres, philosophy, law and government—embarrassing questions sometimes arise as to physicians' general level of intelligence. Whether or not the goodwill and respect of such persons are useful to the medical profession, their contempt is certainly not a comfortable distinction.

But why, it may be asked, should anyone need to learn a writing style from rules and examples? We have all been using language more or less effectively since early childhood. Does a clear thinker and fluent speaker need special training to write well? Yes, he does. In fact, much of the effort of cultivating a satisfactory writing style goes into eradicating habits and modes of expression carried over from speech. Learning to write well consists in large measure in overcoming the handicap of not being able to confront the reader in person and communicate with him vocally.

This point can be illustrated easily by an example. Suppose that you hand a technical paper to an editor, and after reading a page or two he says, "I can't praise this too highly. I'll waste no time in finishing it." His tone, inflection and manner tell you whether he is applauding or condemning your work. Had he dictated the same response to a stenographer, her transcript of his words would leave you in doubt.

The better the writing style, the further it moves from speech style. Characteristically the work of the inexperienced or hurried writer preserves too many of the patterns and conventions of oral communication. As noted elsewhere, spoken and written English are really distinct dialects. In speech, transitions are abrupt and connectives scarce. Words of broad application and vague significance are overworked. Sentence structure is simple and stereotyped but grammatically lax. Syntax is loose and undisciplined, often performing a leap in midsentence. The sequence of ideas may be nearly random. Many expressions are positively incoherent, others wasteful and repetitious. It is not unusual to find a dictated discharge summary in which ten sentences in succession begin, "The patient then. . . ."

Precisely because the diction of well-written English is more self-conscious and artificial than that of speech, it is capable of greater efficiency and economy of expression. Given time for reflection and revision, the writer has the opportunity to express himself much more clearly, vigorously and succinctly than would be possible in speech. Learning to make the best possible use of that opportunity is the very essence of cultivating a writing style.

A major hurdle in one's progress toward an effective style is the need to overcome what we may call the knowledge bias. A writer knows in advance what he is going to say; a reader does not know what he is going to read. Self-evident and banal though this antithesis may seem, it explains many of the worst flaws in substandard technical expression. No one ever mastered the art of writing without learning to see his material through the reader's eye, to view the unfolding of each idea as though it were new to him and as though he did not know what is coming next. When the knowledge bias leads the writer to take too much for granted, communication breaks down and the transmission of ideas falters.

Conquering the knowledge bias, like learning to write orderly and succinct prose, requires breaking habits carried over from speech. A speaker gets immediate visual and auditory cues to tell him whether he is being understood, and unless his hearer's patience runs out he can keep chipping and carving away at his subject until his ideas stand clearly revealed. A writer must achieve the same result with one stroke of the pen. He is entitled to no second chances, and when he tries to snatch them his work grows tedious and repetitious.

A writer can overcome his knowledge bias with practice; he can also revise his writing carefully after letting it become "cold." But the sovereign remedy for the writer's blindness to the reader's blindness is the editor. It is necessary that anyone who undertakes to write for publication have a clear notion of the purpose and function of an editor. Editing has several meanings, only two of which concern us here:

1. Selecting material for publication, directing the mechanics of publication, or more simply publishing. This kind of editing is performed by an editor-in-chief, a senior editor or a publisher, who decides whether a piece of writing is worth printing and if it meets criteria and standards set up for his journal or publishing firm. After tentatively accepting a paper for publication the editor may suggest changes in its length, scope, organization or tone.

2. Copyediting: preparing a text for publication by correcting errors of form (spelling, grammar) and standardizing mechanical features (punctuation, abbreviations). The copyeditor is a patient and resourceful alchemist who transmutes the writer's lead into gold. Copyediting is an

indispensable preliminary to printing, for even when the copyeditor cannot find any errors to correct—and he always can—he has to supply directions to the printer regarding type faces and sizes, format, spacing and the like. This is the copyeditor's special province and is best left entirely to him. Because the other side of copyediting, the improvement of syntax, is a sensitive issue with writers, particularly beginning ones, it merits some discussion.

In order to explain what happens during textual editing, it may be best to start by showing what editing is not. One can edit another's essay or novel, but not another's painting or sculpture. An artist is credited, rightly or wrongly, with a special and unique vision, and accorded the right to interpret it in his own unique fashion. Shapes, colors, textures—the symbols of his "language"—have no conventional meanings: the artist himself works out their meanings in the act of creating and combining them.

A writer is in a different position altogether, for though his vision may well be unique, his words and his manner of putting them together must not be. Admittedly some writers—Edward Lear and Lewis Carroll, François Rabelais and James Joyce—have used language in a way that transcends the literal and strictly conventional function of words while retaining a strong dependence on that function. Their work, like paintings and statues, could almost be said to defy editing.

Carroll, in *Through the Looking-Glass,* wrote the following oft-quoted exchange:

"When *I* use a word," Humpty Dumpty said, in rather a
scornful tone, "it means just what I choose it to mean—
neither more nor less."
"The question is," said Alice, "whether you *can* make words
mean so many different things."
"The question is," said Humpty Dumpty, "which is to be
master—that's all."

Alas for literary ambition and creativity, it is neither the word nor the worker in words who is the real master, but the reader. And the watchdog who looks out for the reader's interests, picking and pawing over the writer's work like a kind of devil's advocate, searching for blunders and discrepancies and passages of confusion and nonsense, is the copyeditor. If there is even a chance that a reader may stumble over a passage, the editor is there to stumble over it first and then mend it.

Editing so often means excising that in the writer's view it may take on a predominantly negative connotation, as he sees his favorite adjectives deleted and his most exuberant flights of fancy recast in more conventional molds. But a good editor is a coadjutor to be appreciated and cherished, not the meddlesome nincompoop that he may seem to the fledgling writer. Trust the editor just as you expect your patient to trust you when you tell him that one of his favorite organs must come out.

There must never be rancor between writer and editor. The editor himself would be the first to admit that his own writing is as much in need of editing as anyone else's. Every writer has stylistic idiosyncrasies that vex and perplex every reader but himself. Even toward those flaws of which he is aware he may be too indulgent a parent if left to his own devices. It takes a writer with the faith of Abraham to follow Sir Arthur Quiller-Couch's advice regarding florid and overblown phraseology: "Murder your darlings."

Not all medical editors are of the same stamp, and not all are equally suited to their work. The physician-turned-editor often has a blind spot regarding linguistic purity and elegance. He may, for example, justify the most outrageous errors in medical Latin and the most flagrant breaches of usage on the grounds that no one would be likely to misunderstand them. The nonphysician who functions as a medical editor, abstracter or translator often falls into glaring technical errors through undue reliance on medical dictionaries and other general references—and, I need hardly add, by failing to recognize inaccuracies and obscurities in the original material. The truly skillful editor works with a scalpel, not an axe. He can refine all but the most slovenly manuscripts with a few deft alterations and sparing deletions. He has learned the lesson that a coarse file never leaves a fine finish. Most of the outstanding medical editors of the present century have been gifted writers themselves.

It might seem that the availability of such talent and ingenuity obviates the need for care and application in writing. After all, if the editor is so good at his job why should the medical writer take the trouble to write clearly and well? By the same reasoning, one should ignore his health completely and let the doctor worry about what to do if he gets sick. The editor is a catalyst, not an equal partner; the chief responsibility for the content and style of writing rests with the author.

More to the point, an editor may believe that there is not enough good material in a garbled and slipshod manuscript to repay the effort of extraction and refining. He may not even be able to tell what the writer is trying to say. Most professional editors are remarkably astute, but they are not mind readers. An ounce of good writing is worth a pound of editing. A very rough manuscript, containing many words and phrases needing emendation and hence offering many opportunities for variation, may diverge sharply from the author's intended meaning by the time that it has been thoroughly edited. Even a skillful editor may not be able to salvage a badly botched manuscript. (Then, too, even an inept editor will probably not be able to ruin a well-written one.)

Joint authorship may eliminate some of the work of the editor, but of course nothing can actually be written by more than one person. Literary collaborators write alternate chapters of their novels, not alternate words. Nevertheless, discussing what has been written with a co-worker will often bring to light omissions, obscurities and absurdities which an editor might have let pass. But no amount of discussion, and no intervention of the professional editor, can substitute for doing a good job of writing in the first place. The proficient and successful writer is his own first editor and most exacting critic.

Self-editing is one of the most crucial and difficult skills in the craft of authorship. Writing is a creative art, and nothing so cramps the artistic spirit or stifles originality as regulation and regimentation. But in technical communication, as in poetry, fiction and drama, fertility must be tempered by judgment, and the faculty of invention by stern self-criticism.

No one can use language effectively without observing the semantic and syntactic conventions that form the subject matter of grammar. Admittedly the classical authors did not compose their words according to the rules of primitive grammarians—quite the reverse. But precisely because the rules of grammar do formulate what is most salutary and useful about the conventions of prose composition, these rules must be observed by anyone who wishes to produce writing that can be understood, appreciated and enjoyed.

A grammatical rule covers all contingencies. It saves the writer the trouble of judging, perhaps wrongly, whether a construction is clear. More importantly, it establishes a principle according to which the reader can interpret quickly and confidently what he reads. In this light, grammatical conventions may be viewed as an outgrowth of the conventions regarding the meanings of words.

Common sense and the example of established patterns of language are useful but by no means infallible guides to good usage. Though we all learn to put the grammatical rules of our native tongue into practice before we learn the rules themselves, no one can produce writing of high quality by merely observing rules. True mastery of language depends on a rational understanding of its patterns, its potentials and its limitations. Moreover, an orderly and objective discussion of style is impossible without recourse to the nomenclature of descriptive grammar. Accordingly, in the next two chapters I present, as succinctly as possible, a survey of English accidence, syntax and punctuation. Succeeding chapters will take up the fundamentals of style.

Although the mechanics of preparing a manuscript for editing lie outside the scope of this book, a few basic recommendations are in order. Every manuscript submitted for publication should be professionally typewritten, double-spaced, on only one side of each sheet. Select a good quality of 8½" x 11" white typewriter bond. Though second-rate typists are naturally fond of "erasable" paper, editors abhor it because the writing on it smears with handling.

Generous margins should be left above, below and on both sides of the typewritten text. Remember that the end product of your efforts is just raw material to the copyeditor. Follow to the letter the publisher's editorial guidelines regarding manuscript preparation. These are generally printed in at least some numbers of a journal as *Directions for* (or *Advice to*) *Authors*. Among the references listed at the end of this chapter are several sources of information on editorial standards for manuscript preparation and bibliographic styling.

Carefully review the typed manuscript for errors. If you must make extensive corrections or changes, have the affected pages retyped. Number all pages in sequence from cover-sheet through bibliography but do not bind or staple them together. Send your manuscript by first-class mail and be sure to keep a photographic or carbon copy. Enclose return postage if you expect the manuscript to be returned to you in case of rejection.

THE CULTIVATION OF STYLE

To say of a surgeon that he is a good technician, and to say no more, is to damn him with faint praise. Though every surgeon aspires to good technique, a good surgeon is more than a mere technician, for besides mechanical skill he possesses mental dexterity, diagnostic acumen, sound judgment, coolheadedness, courage and optimism.

A good writer must go far beyond the punctilious observance of grammatical rules. He must be more than an apt pupil. In writing as in surgery, excellence depends on a due blending of science and art, of the mechanical with the intellectual and the esthetic.

What is style? The word has at least three meanings that we do not want here. When we speak of Osler's style we mean a certain person's conscious language practices. If we say that something is done with style we refer to flair, individuality and orginality in its execution. To the editor and the publisher style means consistency in the mechanics of writing—in grammar, spelling, punctuation and the other standards formulated in a so-called style manual.

The style with which we are concerned here is the technique or practice of expressing ideas accurately, clearly, concisely, and in an order and manner appropriate to the subject. Style in this sense takes mechanical grammar as its point of departure and soon leaves it far behind. Unfortunately it is much easier to recognize a bad style, and to say why it is bad, than to identify with precision the marks of a good one. In broad terms we may list the traits of good formal technical writing as accuracy, organization, clarity and readability. Each of these depends in some measure on the others, and each ought to be in evidence at every level of writing: words, sentences, paragraphs, chapters or sections, and the piece as a whole.

Techniques for achieving clarity, succinctness and coherence cannot be reduced to rules of general and almost automatic application like the principles of grammar. The writer on style must be content to state some guiding principles both positive and negative, illustrate them with a few well-chosen examples, and leave the reader to do the rest for himself. Most of the remaining chapters of this book are devoted to those principles and examples. Here I wish to offer some reflections on two priceless means of cultivating a style that lie within everyone's reach: reading and practice.

Ingelfinger attributes much of the turgidity and raggedness of modern medical writing to the failure of physicians to read nonmedical literature. (Ingelfinger FJ: "Obfuscation" in medical writing. *NEJM* 294:546-547, 1976.) The average American physician probably does less leisure reading than the average bluecollar worker. Stultified by overwork and the demands of an exacting and exhausting vocation, the physician is apt to seek more physical diversions in moments of leisure, and to shun the intellectual challenges of literature.

It is not, of course, a question of how much one reads, or how attentively and docilely, but of the quality of the reading matter. We live in an era of stylistic decadence in which it is hard to find a middle ground between the deadly dullness of the savant and the undisciplined fireworks of the popular novelist, between the bland banalities of the journalist and the impenetrable gibberish of the civil servant. Part of the blame lies with the public, whose insatiable but uncritical demand for reading matter annually calls forth millions of tons of facile, sleazy claptrap; part of it lies with our system of education, which annually sends forth thousand of high-school graduates who can barely read and write. (The educator's postmortem diagnosis for these wretched victims of his incompetence is "functional illiteracy.")

Neither modern literature nor modern education is my subject, and I cannot stop to mourn the tragic plight of either. Suffice it to say that not everything that appears in print is a fitting model for the apprentice writer. Some discrimination is in order. An ear jaded and corrupted, and perhaps slightly deafened, by the stark inanities of rock music struggles in vain to appreciate the intricate counterpoint of Bach or the lush harmonies of Franck. A mind poisoned by the crude babel of cheap fiction and numbed by the relentelss cacophony of journalese may overlook all that is wholesome and commendable in the work of exemplary writers.

To prescribe a reading diet for the aspiring writer, listing authors permitted and authors forbidden, would be to venture into the perilous waters of literary criticism, where I would very soon be beyond my depth. Any reader with a little judgment can select for himself writers whose prose diction is consistently simple, exact and appealing. Reading for instruction in composition and style ought not to be approached as a necessary but distasteful task. Literature from which you recoil in boredom and confusion will scarecely be a fitting model for the cultivation of your own style.

On no account should you waste your time trying to pick up pointers on style by reading a book whose subject does not interest you. Matter and form are too intimately interdependent for such an exercise to yield much benefit. Outstanding stylists write in every genre of prose literature. It is unnecessary to confine yourself to nonfiction, and imprudent to stay within the present century. Much can be learned from the great novelists and essayists of the eighteenth and nineheenth centuries, though I would not advise the technical writer to copy Gibbon's majestic but soporific phraseology or Lamb's mellifluous but eccentric prose.

When Sir William Osler prepared his list of (nonmedical) books that should be on every medical student's shelf, he was evidently concerned with the formation of mind and character, not with writing style. For example, his list includes the *Essais* of Montaigne, whose highly spontaneous and richly figurative language, with its sudden transitions and total lack of organization, would hardly be a suitable model for the scientific writer. But Osler also recommended Ralph Waldo Emerson and Oliver Wendell Holmes, two American essayists from whom no earnest and discriminating technical writer should scorn to take lessons. Holmes' reputation as a poet and essayist have thrown his medical career into the shadow. Let it not be forgotten that he wrote about the contagiousness of puerperal fever before Semmelweis, coined the term *anesthetic,* and was known in his day as so astute a scientific reasoner that his British colleague and junior, Arthur Conan Doyle, named the incomparable Sherlock after him.

In his introduction to an edition of Osler's collected papers, Dr. Paul Dudley White added Osler's own works, both technical and literary, to the famous reading list. (See White PD: Introduction, in Osler W: *Aequanimitas and Other Papers,* New York, W W Norton & Co, Inc, 1963.) Osler had studied briefly for the ministry before turning to medicine, and it has been suggested that his familiarity with the rich and vigorous idiom of the English Bible (which also appears on his list) and the Episcopal Prayer Book contributed to the formation of his own lucid, supple and sinewy style, the envy and despair of the modern medical writer. The neophyte who seeks inspiration and example need look no further than Osler's *Principles and Practice of Medicine,* which is both a masterpiece of English prose and a monument to the brilliance of the author as a clinician, scientist and teacher. This work, which went through eighteen editions, is now long out of print, and even the later revisions have the demerit of being technically obsolete. A generous and representative sample of Osler's medical writing, together with valuable commentary, can be found in Harvey AM, McKusick V (eds): *Osler's Textbook Revisited,* New York, Appleton-Century-Crofts, 1967.

Among earlier scientific writers Charles Darwin and Thomas Huxley may be offered as models. Darwin once asserted that the whole credit for making a discovery ought to go to the man who succeeded in impressing it on the minds of his readers. Though he was not then talking about his own work, *The Origin of Species,* the remark applies with perfect accuracy to that milestone in the history of science. The book is a *tour de force* of technical exposition, a brilliant mosaic of description, narration, experimental reporting, analysis, demonstration, induction and documentation. By the sheer weight of its evidence and the flawless integrity of its logic, it forced the scientific world to accept the theory of natural selection despite all the opposition that dogmatism, prejudice and ignorance could muster.

Darwin's style has been sharply criticized, from his day to ours, as being ambiguous, convoluted and generally obscure. Certainly his powers of organizing and analyzing facts surpassed his ability to state them in crisp, lucid, sprightly English. But though he is more honored as an observer and thinker than as a writer, it was not merely his concept of natural selection (which was not original with him) or even the evidence he accumulated in support of it (much of which has been proved false or irrelevant) that changed the whole course of modern science, but his singlehanded statement of his case in *The Origin of Species.* For this reason Darwin holds a special place in the history of technical writing and the reader must be prepared to excuse me for introducing later in the book two or three passages of his stodgy Victorian prose.

Darwin's friend and advocate, Thomas Huxley, was a naturalist and physician who published numerous scientific communications in a style conspicuous for its vigor, directness and clarity. Many of his most important works on "natural history" were directed at a lay audience. With his scientific genius and literary flair he revealed to ordinary people the wonders of nature and popularized the developing science of his day, much as Buffon had done in France a century earlier. (Buffon is remembered nowadays chiefly for his *Discourse on Style,* wherein appears the famous dictum, "Style is of the man himself"—that is, is personal or individual—often misquoted or mistranslated as "Style is the man himself.")

More modern authors whose technical writing styles commend themselves include Harvey Cushing, William Halsted, Philip Thorek, Sir Zachary Cope and Harry Beckman. Many others might be mentioned. I do not suggest that the aspiring medical writer "play the sedulous ape" to these authors, as Stevenson confessed doing to Hazlitt, Lamb and Wordsworth. What I propose is not a conscious imitation of the vocabulary, phrasing or manner of any one writer, but a gradual and painless absorption, from the example of many good writers, of the principles of orderly, clear, concise and readable exposition.

In comparing the two passages which follow, we are struck by the extreme contrast of spirit and tone as well as by differences in vocabulary and syntax. The first specimen, an excerpt from Osler's *Principles and Practice of Medicine,* derives its character not only from the author's perfect mastery of both subject and language, but also from his evident intention to write sound and sober sense. Whatever motivated the author of the second passage, it cannot have been solely a desire to express himself in plain, vigorous and direct language:

> We know but little of the incubation period in acute lobar pneumonia. It is probably very short. There are sometimes slight catarrhal symptoms for a day or two. As a rule, the disease sets in abruptly with a severe chill, which lasts from fifteen to thirty minutes or longer. In no acute disease is an initial chill so constant or so severe. The patient may be taken abruptly in the midst of his work, or may awaken out of a sound sleep in a rigor. The temperature taken during the chill shows that the fever has already begun. If seen shortly after the onset, the patient has usually features of an acute fever, and complains of headache and general pains. Within a few hours there is pain in the side, often of an agonizing character; a short, dry, painful cough begins, and the respirations are increased in frequency. When seen on the second or third day, the picture in typical pneumonia is more distinctive than that presented by any other acute disease. The patient lies flat in bed, often on the affected side; his face is flushed, particularly one or both cheeks; the breathing is hurried, accompanied often with a short expiratory grunt; the alae nasi dilate with each inspiration; herpes is usually present on the lips or nose; the eyes

are bright, the expression is anxious, and there is a frequent short cough which makes the patient wince and hold his side. The expectoration is blood-tinged and extremely tenacious. The temperature may be 104° or 105°. The pulse is full and bounding and the pulse-respiration ratio much disturbed. Examination of the lungs shows the physical signs of consolidation—blowing breathing and fine rales. After persisting for from seven to ten days the crisis occurs, and with a fall in the temperature the patient passes from the condition of extreme distress and anxiety to one of comparative comfort. (Osler W: *The Principles and Practice of Medicine,* ed 9. New York, D Appleton & Co, 1909, article "Lobar Pneumonia.")

Symptomatology relative to impending or incipient onset of illness generally manifests itself initially via a marked chill, following which a rapid rise of temperature to the 103° - 105° range is characteristically observed. Cutaneous palpation demonstrates evidence of considerable warmth and dryness, while erythema of the malar eminences accompanies fever in a majority of instances. The facies is furthermore characterized by an expression of anxiety, with alar flaring occurring synchronously with inspiratory activity. There are usually also cephalgia, myalgia, severe thirst, marked anorexia and other constitutional manifestations commonly attendant upon any febrile condition, as well as tachycardia, with pulse substantially higher than 100, and tachypnea with respiratory frequency exceeding sometimes 60 per minute. Within a 24-hour period after acute symptom onset a sensation of moderate to marked distress incident on development of acute inflammation of the pleural membrane investing the particular part of the lung in which the pneumonic process has established itself generally makes itself known and in the generality of cases is pleuritic in character, i.e., lancinating, sharply localized and precipitated by inspiratory movements though not altogether abolished by temporary cessation of breathing activity, in spite of the fact that both voluntary and involuntary partial immobilization, i.e., splinting of the side of the thorax involved is the rule rather than the exception. Cough with production of tenacious and often frankly sanguineous or sanguineopurulent expectoration generally commences at about the same point of time as pleuritic pain, and as would be anticipated aggravates pleuritic distress, the patient therefore endeavoring to suppress both the frequency and the intensity of tussive efforts.

I submit that anyone accustomed to reading literature, whether technical or not, of the tone and calibre of the first paragraph would be virtually incapable of writing rubbish like the second.

"Reading maketh a full man," wrote Bacon, but he presently added, "and writing an exact man." Judicious and attentive reading cannot by itself foster the ability to write well. The most accomplished writer is not the most voracious or even the most tenacious reader but the most resolute and indomitable scribbler. By the sweat on his brow, the ink on his fingers, and the litter of discarded drafts on his floor you may measure both his determination and his progress in the art of verbal expression.

The avoidance of jingles, miscues and dangling modifiers must become a conditioned reflex, as the writer repeatedly puts himself into the reader's position, listening, testing, weighing alternatives. Though these techniques may seem to become second nature as the writer grows proficient, no part of his craft can be permitted to become routine. The writer who believes that it can will be a pedestrian stylist just as surely as the physician whose examination of the abdomen is a perfunctory and unvarying ritual will be an inept diagnostician. Routine and method are not the same thing.

Practice in writing may take various forms. Its end product need not be a finished paper suitable for publication. A valuable means of refining your style is to take something published by someone else and try to make it better: find a more exact word, a more direct construction, a shorter, more distinctive, more pleasing way of narrating, describing or explaining. Nothing in print is so perfect that it cannot be improved. However, finding flaws to correct in the work of a particularly accomplished writer is a job for a particularly skillful (or captious) editor. (The present volume should provide ample scope for the beginner.)

A second way of using another writer's material to sharpen your own skills is preparing abstracts of technical papers, or of anything you like. Not only does this practice train you to clarify and condense language to its quintessential elements, but if you work with papers in your special field of interest it will broaden your knowledge of the pertinent literature and provide you with a collection of highly compressed reference materials. When you have reduced the material to its smallest compass, count the words, tear up your abstract, and start over with a limit of just half as many words as before.

Opportunities for practice are ever-present for the physician who wants to develop his ability to write on clinical subjects with clarity, precision and vigor. Instead of relegating the preparation of reports and correspondence to underlings, tackle these jobs yourself, with the goal of producing material that would be fit for publication. Instead of grinding out dictated reports full of banal formulas and disorganized rambling, take the time to collect and arrange your thoughts, and make your words and phrases as accurate, felicitous and distinctive as you can.

Many a clinical instructor who can speak lucidly and succinctly on ward rounds or in a seminar deteriorates into a gibbering numbskull when he takes pen in hand. For some the act of writing paralyzes the intellect and dams up the stream of ideas, so that simple matters become tangled, turgid and obscure. If you have such a problem, you can teach yourself an unforgettable lesson in prose composition by turning your back on pen and paper and expressing your thoughts to a dictating machine or tape recorder. The simplicity, directness and precision of the playback may astound you.

Besides all the other qualities of a competent technical writer that I have mentioned and shall mention, two stand out in importance: a sense of purpose, and due humility. Truly articulate writing is purposeful writing, and its purpose is evident in every paragraph. Your motive for putting pen to paper should shine forth clearly in the manner and style of your presentation, whether you set out to impart information or defend a thesis. (As an elementary precaution, never start writing unless you have something to say.)

Your real purpose in writing should always be to conquer a problem—ignorance, misinformation, doubt, inadequacy of data—and not an opponent or a whole army of opponents, real or fancied. A contributor to the medical literature is expected to share information or a point of view, not to hand down revelations and pronouncements with Olympian condescension. Arrogance and pugnacity are as unbecoming in a writer as in a physician or scientist. The writer who is not taught humility by his dealings with editors may have a harsher lesson to learn at the hands of readers who disagree with his facts or conclusions, or resent his manner of stating them.

REFERENCES

Davidson HA: *Guide to Medical Writing.* New York, The Ronald Press Co, 1957.
Fishbein M: *Medical Writing: The Technic and the Art,* ed 4. Springfield, Ill, Charles C Thomas, 1972.
Kapp RO: *The Presentation of Technical Information.* New York, Macmillan & Co, 1960.
Meiss HR, Jaeger DA (eds): *Information to Authors: Editorial Guidelines Reprinted from 140 Medical Journals.* New York, Mt Sinai School of Medicine, 1976.

Mitchell JH: *Writing for Professional and Technical Journals.* New York, John Wiley & Sons, Inc, 1968.

O'Leary R: Technic of medical communication. *NEJM* 274:940-944, 1966.

Publication Manual of the American Psychological Association, ed 2. Washington DC, American Psychological Association, 1974.

Stylebook/Editorial Manual of the AMA, ed 6. Littleton, Massachusetts, Publishing Sciences Group, Inc, 1976.

Skillin ME, Gay RM: *Words into Type.* Englewood Cliffs, NJ, Prentice-Hall, Inc, 1974.

Ward RR: *Practical Technical Writing.* New York, Alfred A Knopf, 1968.

4

A Survey of Grammar

I. Substantives, Verbs and Modifiers

This chapter and the next one outline the grammar of English from a predominantly traditional point of view and with traditional nomenclature. To lighten the reader's burden I have kept to the essentials and have often illustrated points of usage with colloquial rather than formal language.

A **word** is the smallest unit of meaning in speech and writing. Words should be spelled, capitalized and pluralized in accordance with current formal usage. (The table on the next page lists some medical terms that are frequently misspelled.)

American spelling should be followed even in translations and in quotations or abstracts of British material. However, Greek and Latin diphthongs should be preserved in titles (*Royal College of Obstetricians and Gynaecologists*), taxonomic terms (*Haemophilus, Entamoeba, N. gonorrhoeae*) and Latin phrases (*placenta praevia, foetor hepaticus*). On this latter point some American medical style manuals disagree.

It would perhaps be best for all concerned if a uniform policy were adopted of pluralizing with -*s* or -*es* any word, regardless of its origin, once it has been taken into use by speakers of English. The few unlovely tongue-twisters that would result from this practice (*epididymises, urinalysises*) would at least be preferable to the bewildering miscellany of plurals presently in use for words of foreign extraction, rendered more motley and chaotic by the exertions of fanatical purists and misinformed

MEDICAL TERMS COMMONLY MISPELLED

Right	Wrong
acneiform	acneform
acrodermatitis	achrodermatitis
aneurysm	aneurism
anhidrosis	anhydrosis
collimator	columnator
desiccate	dessicate
dietitian	dietician
dilatation	dilation
diluent	dilutant
dissecans	dessicans
fundoscopic	funduscopic
gentamicin	gentamycin
hiccup	hiccough
homozygous	homazygous
hypercapnia	hypercapnea
inoculate	innoculate
micturition	micturation
periodontal	peridontal
phalanx	phalynx
plantar (*adjective*)	planter
procidentia	procedentia
rhonchus	ronchus
scabietic	scabetic
sphingomyelin	sphyngomyelin
stilbestrol	stilbesterol
verruca	verucca

pedants. Dreams of linguistic simplicity aside, current usage requires the plurals of many words of Greek and Latin origin to follow the rules of the parent tongue instead of the language of adoption. When in doubt, consult a reliable dictionary.

No one should undertake to write for publication without immediate access to a large English dictionary of recent copyright. A current medical dictionary is indispensable for the medical writer who is not a physician, and nearly so for the one who is. However, a medical dictionary is not necessarily a trustworthy source of information about the meaning of a word, which may have to be found or confirmed in an authoritative textbook or monograph. (See Good R: The doctor and his dictionary. *NEJM* 275:587-590, 1966.)

GROUPS OF WORDS

A **sentence** is a group of words (rarely, a single word) expressing a complete thought. It contains a *subject,* about which something is said or asked, and a *predicate,* which says or asks something about the subject. A sentence begins with a capital letter and ends with a period, a question mark or an exclamation mark. Sentences are divided into four classes.

> DECLARATIVE: He is an asthmatic.
> INTERROGATIVE: How far apart are the pains?
> IMPERATIVE: Swallow several times. (The subject, *you,* is implied but not expressed.)
> EXCLAMATORY: Dash it all, this isn't a needle-holder!

A **phrase** is a group of words that does not express a complete thought because it does not contain both a subject and a predicate.

> another infarct
> in the lymphoid tissue of the small intestine
> were incised and drained

The components of a phrase may be virtually inseparable: *all right, in spite of, The United States of America.* In some cases this semantic fusion has led to physical agglutination: *already, inasmuch, heretofore.*

A **clause** is a group of words that does not stand alone even though it contains both a subject and a predicate. An **independent** or **main clause** could stand by itself, and is distinguished from a sentence only by the fact that it does not do so.

This should correct the acidosis, unless he's in renal failure.

A **dependent** or **subordinate clause** does not express a complete thought but requires the support of an independent clause, whose meaning it in turn amplifies or modifies.

I expected *that the liver function would have reverted to normal by now.*
The patient was a diabetic *whom I had never seen before.*
After he ran out of medicine he gradually slipped back into failure.

An **elliptical clause** is one in which the subject or the predicate has been partly or completely suppressed.

The patient's sister was even sicker than he [was sick].
Warm the solution until [it becomes] perfectly clear.

Sometimes an entire clause is suppressed.

If only we had more time! (Conclusion entirely suppressed.)

A **compound sentence** contains two or more independent clauses.

Proteins and polysaccharides are capable of stimulating antibody formation, and these comprise most of the allergenic substances.

A **complex sentence** contains at least one dependent clause.

Though several theories on SRIF have been proposed, the mechanism of its action is still unknown.

PARTS OF SPEECH

When words and phrases are classified according to their functions in a sentence they are called parts of speech. The eight parts of speech of traditional grammar are noun, pronoun, adjective, verb, adverb, preposition, conjunction and interjection. These terms refer strictly to the function of a word or phrase in a specific sentence, never to its form.

NOUN: Use a large-bore *needle.*
VERB: Were you able to *needle* that cyst?

ADJECTIVE: I'd be in favor of a *needle* biopsy.

ADVERB: If she *but* looks at fiber glass, she breaks out in a rash.

PREPOSITION: He has no one to blame *but* himself.

CONJUNCTION: We were expecting trouble *but* we didn't anticipate a power failure.

Admittedly, the division of word functions into just eight classes oversimplifies language slightly. Some words can act as two parts of speech at once, while others do not fit comfortably into any of the eight groups. Nevertheless this scheme, applied originally to the classical languages, is a highly serviceable tool in the study of English syntax. Though most linguistic reformers have modifed the nomenclature, almost none have abandoned the basic system.

SUBSTANTIVES
(NOUNS AND PRONOUNS)

A **noun** is the name of a person, time, place, thing or quality.

A *pathologist* in another *city* examined the *slides* with great *thoroughness* a *month* ago.

A **proper noun** names a particular person, time, place or thing; its first letter is capitalized.

Mr. Joseph Butters went to *Rochester* on *Monday* for an examination at the *Mayo Clinic.*

All other nouns are **common nouns.** Nouns may also be classified as concrete (*cannula, femur*), abstract (*viscosity, stamina*), collective (*committee, Congress*) and aggregate (*blood, bone*).

The **genitive case** or **form** of a noun denotes possession. The genitive is regularly formed by addition of *'s* to the nominative (uninflected) case. In formal writing, however, this usage is limited to nouns denoting persons or groups of persons (including institutions and countries), animals and plants, buildings, vehicles, times and a few others. With most inanimate objects, *of* is used instead of the *'s* genitive.

After a *month's* delay, the *patient's* records finally arrived in the *hospital's* mail room.

BUT: the sesamoid bones *of the ankle and foot* [NOT *the ankle's and foot's* sesamoid bones]

Besides showing possession, the genitive can express the relation between a person or thing and an action or process. The *subjective genitive* identifies the performer of an action.

> The *surgeon's* refusal to intervene was a purely personal decision.
> BUT: the expansion *of the lung* [NOT *the lung's* expansion]

The *objective genitive* identifies the object of an action.

> The house *staff's* exclusion from the conference was unwise.
> BUT: the removal *of the spleen* [NOT *the spleen's* removal]

A **pronoun** is a word used in place of a noun. The noun which a pronoun represents is called its *antecedent*.

> *He* and *I* thought *it* would be best if *we* saw *her* before *they*
>   brought *you* back.
> *These* are *mine* and *the rest* are *yours*.
> *Some* use estrogen, while *others* prefer androgen; though *the*
> *former* get faster results, *the latter* avoid gastric upset.
> *All* of these lessons are valuable, but *most* of *them* are less so than
>   *those that one* teaches *oneself*.

Pronouns are distinguished as to person and number.

	SINGULAR	PLURAL
FIRST PERSON	I, me	we, us
SECOND PERSON	you	you
THIRD PERSON	he, she, it,	they, them,
	him, her,	these, those
	this, that	

When pronouns of more than one person stand in a series, the proper order is: the person addressed (second person); the person or thing spoken about (third person); the speaker (first person).

> They blame *him and me* for what *you and she* did.
> The parents preferred to discuss it with *you or me*.

Placing a noun in apposition with a pronoun does not require or justify any change in the form of the pronoun.

We Americans can learn much from the experience of the British.
To us general surgeons that method of handling gastric bleeding
    sounds like heresy.

A pronoun must agree with its antecedent in number.

Each patient was instructed to take only the medicines dispensed
    to *him* [NOT *them*].

The interrogative and relative pronouns *who, whose, whom, which* and
what may be either singular or plural. Relative pronouns are discussed in
the next chapter. The possessive pronouns (*my, our, your, his, her, its,
their*) are considered in the section concerning adjectives, since they
properly belong to this class.

The pronoun *it* often serves as an **expletive** in constructions like the
following.

It will come as no surprise that he has peritonitis.
Her general condition makes it necessary that we operate at once.

An expletive is a grammatical orphan which is not strictly speaking any
part of speech, a filler whose removal leaves the meaning intact though it
may require reshuffling of words. Expletives are frequently used in
inverted constructions. The other common expletive is *there*.

There are seven conditions in which propranolol is strongly
    contraindicated.

VERBS

A **verb** is a word or phrase that denotes action or being.

The surgeon *crushed* the pedicle.
By this time tomorrow he *will have been bronchoscoped.*
This aperture *is* the foramen ovale.

The "action" may be purely mental or figurative.

I *wanted* lidocaine but *had* to *settle* for procainamide.

The *subject* of a verb (and of the clause or sentence in which the verb
stands) is that about which the verb says something.

Mr. Roper fell out of bed.
In my judgment the *mass* both looked and felt malignant.

A verb must agree with its subject in number, that is, if the subject is singular the verb must also be singular, and if the subject is plural the verb must be plural. A subject is plural when it is a single substantive denoting more than one (*they, lungs, media*) or a group of substantives (*prostaglandin E and angiotensin*). Ensuring agreement of subject and verb requires special care when the words stand apart, or in inverted order.

An extensive proliferation of fibroblasts, small round cells and giant cells *was* [NOT *were*] found in the area of the injury.
There *are* [NOT *is*] loss of normal architecture, foci of hyalinized and acellular collagen and replacement of the fibrosa with myxomatous tissue.

The pronouns *each, either, neither* and *none* take singular verbs in formal writing.

On radiographic examination neither of the vessels *was* [COLLOQUIAL: *were*] patent.

When the subject has a collective significance its meaning rather than its form may determine the number of the verb.

A *variety* of useful procedures *have* been developed.
Twelve hundred *calories is* about the lowest maintenance limit for an active adult.

Though *a number, a variety, a combination* and the like often take a plural verb, any of these words preceded by *the, this* or *that* takes a singular verb.

A combination of causes have interacted to produce an irreversible acidosis.
BUT: This combination of clinical findings has been observed primarily in Japanese children.

When a verb has two subjects, one singular and one plural, separated by *or* or *nor,* the verb agrees in number with the subject nearer to it.

Neither the liver nor the *kidneys were* involved.
Neither the kidneys nor the *liver was* involved.

Connecting phrases like *as well as, together with* and *but also* lack the full force of *and.* Accordingly, a singular subject followed by such a phrase ordinarily takes a singular verb.

> The pituitary-adrenal axis, in concert with the autonomic nervous system, exercises a profound influence on resting arterial pressure.

An *object* or *complement* explains or completes the idea expressed by a verb. (However, not every sentence contains a complement.) The action denoted by a **transitive verb** takes a **direct object.**

	TR. VERB.	DIR. OBJ.
A bone fragment	*penetrated*	*the spleen.*

An **intransitive verb** takes no object.

> My chest *hurts* when I *inhale.*

Many verbs can be either transitive or intransitive.

> The fractured rib *tore* the spleen.
> The spleen *tore.*

A verb that denotes giving, sending or offering may take an **indirect object** as well as a direct one. The indirect object is often introduced by *to.*

> The vagus supplies sensory and motor fibers to *thoracic and abdominal viscera.*
> Hand *me* that towel. OR Hand that towel to *me.*

The verb and its complement, if any, compose the **predicate** of the sentence.

> All of the cultures in that third batch *died.*
> He *refused to follow directions and even told the nurse that his father had taken off his dressing and thrown away his clindamycin.*

A **copulative verb,** which denotes being or becoming, does not take a direct object; neither does a **descriptive verb** such as *seem, appear, feel, taste, smell.* A copulative or descriptive verb affirms or denies the identity or equivalence of two terms. When its complement is a substantive it is called a *predicate nominative.*

>The liver is not a hollow *viscus.*

A **factitive verb** (denoting thinking, calling, appointing and the like) may take both a direct object and an *oblique complement.*

DIR. OBJ.   OBL. COMP.

>We had no choice but to appoint   *Dr. Richter   chief of surgery.*

When the subject performs the action denoted by the verb, the verb is said to be in the **active voice.**

>The patient *slipped* on the throw-rug, *fell* against the edge of the open door, *fractured* her left zygomatic arch and *bruised* her left shoulder.

When the subject receives the action the verb is in the **passive voice.**

>The patient *was intubated* without difficulty.
>This vessel *is obstructed* just above the bifurcation.

Only a transitive verb can become passive. Normally a passive verb does not take any complement, but an exception may occur with a passive verb denoting giving or offering. When the substantive that would otherwise be the indirect object of such a verb becomes its subject (*Baker* was given a medal), the direct object appears as a complement, the so-called *retained object* (Baker was given a *medal*). The oblique complement of a factitive verb may also become a retained object.

>She was elected *director* by a large majority.

The **tense** of a verb, broadly speaking, establishes a temporal relation between the action indicated and the moment at which the verb is uttered.

>PAST: We *found* a solitary cyst in the left kidney.
>PRESENT: Diabetic retinopathy *is* evident here.
>FUTURE: Only time *will tell.*

The perfect tenses refer to actions already completed.

PAST PERFECT: They *had* already *tied* off the superior thyroid
artery.

PRESENT PERFECT: I *have reviewed* all the autopsy material

FUTURE PERFECT: He *will have had* seven dilatations by Thursday.

All of the perfect tenses, as well as the simple future, are compound
or phrasal tenses formed with auxiliary verbs such as *has, had* and *will.*
These and other auxiliary verbs, including *am, is, are, was, were, be, been,*
being, do, did and *done,* enter into a variety of verbal constructions.

PROGRESSIVE TENSES (with participle): We *have been* having a lot of
trouble with the phase microscope.

NEGATION (with *not*): These tumors *do* not often metastasize to
bone.

QUESTIONS: *Did* you notice his tremor?

PASSIVE VOICE: The joints which *had been* affected longest *were* in-
jected first.

Classical grammar, based on Greek and Latin, distinguishes several
moods or **modes** of the verb. The *indicative mood* states a fact.

The left calyx *is* normal.

The *imperative mood* gives a command.

Turn your head and *cough.*

The *subjunctive mood* expresses conditions, possibilities, probabilities,
necessities and wishes. In English it is formed almost exclusively with the
modal auxiliary verbs *may, can, might, could, should, would, must,*
ought and a few others.

If he *should fibrillate,* the monitor *would alert* you.

This *may hurt* a little.

This is the first such reaction I have seen; *may* it *be* the last.

Most of the subjunctives formed without modal auxiliaries are now
nearly obsolete (If this *be* treason . . . ; Ah! wilderness *were* paradise
enow.). However, there are some exceptions which must be carefully
observed in formal writing.

When a conditional clause expresses a condition that is contrary to
fact, its verb must be in the subjunctive mood.

If he *were* twenty years younger, we could operate at once.

When a condition is not necessarily contrary to fact, the indicative mood is used.

If he *is* on digitalis, he's getting either too little or too much.

When a subordinate clause expresses a thought, wish, demand or requirement, formal usage distinguishes it from a statement of fact by using a subjunctive verb.

It is neither desirable nor necessary that he *be subjected* to general anesthesia.
They asked that he *take* the oral examination in April.

English makes less extensive use of subjunctive verb forms than classical (and many modern) languages. Ordinarily the indicative mood is preferred in indirect questions and in subordinate clauses other than those mentioned above.

They wanted to know if I *was* [NOT *were*] on call Monday night.
Initial application of cold is appropriate for all soft tissue
injuries, whether they *are* [NOT *be*] burns, contusions,
sprains or muscle pulls.

Subjunctive verb forms survive in a few set phrases: as it *were, be* that as it may.

MODIFIERS
(AJECTIVES)

An **adjective** is a word or phrase that modifies (qualifies, amplifies, describes or limits) a noun or pronoun. The substantive which an adjective modifies is called its *headword*. Articles (*a, an, the*) and possessive pronouns (*my, our, your, his, her, its, their*) are adjectives. The *'s* genitive form of a noun may also be thought of as an adjective.

Both the common bile duct and *the cystic* duct immediately *adjacent* to it were *edematous.*

The normal position of an adjective is before its headword. A few headwords (*something, anyone*) are regularly followed by their adjectives.

There is something peculiar about these data.

Sometimes placement of an adjective after its headword improves clarity and readability.

I suspect a condition different from the one you mentioned.
A second urine specimen, sterile and freshly voided, was obtained
next morning.

Note that in the first example it would be awkward to separate the adjective from the words following it. In the second example the two adjectives following their headword are set off by commas because they are descriptive, not essential. They are said to be in loose apposition with *specimen.* Since in the first example *different* defines or specifies its headword, it is not set off by commas.

A copulative, descriptive or factitive verb may take an adjective as its complement. Such a complement is called a *predicate adjective.*

The patient appears *older* than his stated age.
Unfortunately your hypothesis proved *correct.*
Hold the hand *flat* and *horizontal.*

When a noun is used unchanged as an attributive adjective, as in *heart block* and *skin graft,* only its position before another noun indicates its function. Such a noun should not ordinarily be turned into a predicate adjective.

*The rhythm was *sinus.*

The article may be omitted before a noun which is used in a general or abstract way.

Urine normally contains only a negligible quantity of conjugated
bilirubin.
BUT: The urine was grossly bloody and contained many granular
casts.

Though usage is divided, in formal writing it is generally appropriate, and sometimes necessary, to repeat an article before each member of a

*Here, as elsewhere throughout this book, the asterisk indicates a specimen of faulty usage.

pair or longer series, provided that the first article is not followed by an adjective which modifies every member of the series.

> the liver, the spleen and the lymph nodes
> the liver, the spleen and the enlarged lymph nodes
> the enlarged liver, the spleen and the lymph nodes (Only the liver is enlarged.)
> BUT: the enlarged liver, spleen and lymph nodes (All are enlarged.)

There are many exceptions to this principle, some of them dictated by usage and some by the ear. The article is often omitted when the members of the series are thought of as a unit, and nearly always when they are in fact identical.

> Last week he had an incision and drainage [NOT an incision and a drainage].
> Dr. Lorenz has a high reputation as a writer and editor [NOT as a writer and an editor].

Nouns separated by *or* or *nor* less often require repetition of the article. The article should usually be repeated, however, when a sharp distinction is expressed, particularly after *either, neither* or *whether.*

> A retractor or other heavy instrument can be as dangerous a weapon as a scalpel.
> Deformity is often more apparent to the physician than to the parents or siblings of the patient.
> BUT: We had no way of knowing whether it was a neoplasm or *an* abscess.

Comparative ("more") and superlative ("most") forms of adjectives are generally made with the suffixes *-er* and *-est*. Exceptions include a few irregular comparatives and superlatives (*better, best; worse, worst; less, least,* etc.) and adjectives that are regularly compared by the adverbs *more* and *most* to avoid awkwardness.

> more edematous, most edematous; NOT edematouser, edematousest

Not all cases in which good usage demands *more* and *most* are as obvious as this. When in doubt, consult a dictionary.

An **adverb** is a word or phrase that modifies a verb, an adjective or another adverb.

The patient died *suddenly.*
The risk of complications is *exceedingly* remote.
These tissues *almost never* regenerate.
Of course, it will take *at least* a week.

Many adverbs have been formed from adjectives by the addition of the suffix *-ly.* Colloquial usage allows "flat" adverbs ("He held on tight"; "It's coming down slow"), but in formal writing the *-ly* form is nearly always expected. (*Muchly* and *thusly,* however, are vulgarisms.) A flat adverb is perfectly acceptable in formal usage when it differs in meaning from the *-ly* form.

Dr. Bray dispenses penicillin *freely.*
Dr. Bray dispenses penicillin *free.*

Comparative and superlative forms of *-ly* adverbs are made with *more* and *most.* Other adverbs are generally compared like adjectives.

Hysterostomatotomy is *more easily* [COLLOQUIAL: *easier*] done than
   said.
The pressure kept rising *faster.*

The position of an adverb with respect to its headword is much more variable than that of an adjective.

The first treatment *completely* destroyed the lesion.
The first treatment destroyed the lesion *completely.*

Variation in the position of the adverb may produce a shift, often subtle, in meaning.

Only the creatinine declined slightly with hydration.
The creatinine declined *only* slightly with hydration.
The creatinine declined slightly with hydration *only.*

Though colloquial usage allows considerable latitude in the position of an adverb, in writing it must be so placed that its bearing is immediately clear.

*The patient only reported pinkish sputum yesterday.

This should be recast to show which of the following meanings is intended.

Only the patient reported pinkish sputum yesterday. (No one else
did.)
The patient reported only pinkish sputum yesterday. (—but not
gross hemoptysis.)
The patient reported pinkish sputum only yesterday. (—but not
before.)

It is sometimes impossible to identify with certainty the headword of
an adverb. In some cases the adverb may be said to modify an entire
clause or sentence.

Admittedly, overnight storage of inoculated medium in the
refrigerator does not enhance the yield of pathogens.

A sentence adverb may be moved almost anywhere without much change
in meaning. In the following sentence, *perhaps* could be inserted at any
of the carets.

∧ Of all the cells in the body ∧ the myocardial and brain cells ∧
show ∧ a greater dependency on aerobic metabolism than ∧
any other.

Adverbs can act as conjunctions by introducing or connecting clauses.
(Conjunctions are discussed in the next chapter.)

The prothrombin time was fifty-one seconds; *accordingly* liver
biopsy was not done.
Once he has overcome his addiction to pizza his recovery should
be rapid and uneventful.

Sometimes the distinction between adjective and adverb is difficult to
make. The following principles should help to clarify the difference.
1. When a copulative or descriptive verb is followed by a single
modifier, that modifier must be a predicate adjective and not an adverb.

On the subject of peer review Dr. Pavon waxed [=became]
eloquent [NOT *eloquently*].
You forgot to ask how long the patient has been feeling *bad* [NOT
badly].

2. Any intransitive verb may take a predicate adjective if its purport is
mainly descriptive.

Children should be urged not to walk *barefoot* in the grass.

The patient's brother dropped *dead* at the age of 41, and an uncle is reported to have died even *younger.*

The choice between adjective and adverb may be arbitrary.

Hope springs *eternal* OR *eternally.*

The urethra ended *blind* OR *blindly.*

5

A Survey of Grammar

II. Connectives, Relative Clauses,

Verbals and Punctuation

Connectives are the nails and screws, the handles and signposts of language. They seem far less important than other parts of speech until we try to do without them, or fall into habits of using them incorrectly.

A **preposition** introduces a substantive word or phrase and shows how it is related to some other part of the sentence. The substantive which it introduces is called its *object*. A phrase consisting of a preposition and its object usually functions as an adjective or an adverb.

> ADJECTIVE: An infant *in respiratory distress* may appear normal
>   until respirations are counted.
> ADVERB: The liver cannot function *without oxygen*.

A preposition may be a phrase: *according to, because of, distal to, in order to*. Some prepositions have been adapted from other parts of speech: *regarding, including, except*. Though these examples are old and firmly established as prepositions, others of more recent date (*following, previous to, due to*) are objectionable to language purists, chiefly because they are new. Careful writers avoid them not so much for that reason as because their new functions and meanings have not altogether displaced

73

the old, so that they may be imprecise or ambiguous. These points are discussed further in Chapter 10.

Almost the only inviolate rule of word order in Latin is that a preposition must always come before its object. Indeed, this part of speech gets its name not from its function but from its constant position (*praepositum = placed before*). Traditional English grammarians clung so stubbornly to this rule of syntax that they condemned all such natural expressions as "What is the world coming to?" and "I see what you're driving at," in which the prepositions do not stand in front of anything.

Early in this century, professional educators finally admitted that these constructions were ineradicable from the common speech. They gave up trying to get rid of them and salved their consciences with the harmless but absurd fiction that the caboose prepositions are adverbs. In a few constructions, such as "Nowadays such lesions are seldom met with," the designation of the last word as an adverb is plausible, if not incontrovertible. But in "the practice which I most strenuously object to," the last word is clearly a preposition which both speaker and hearer feel is more closely related to the verb than to its object. Though modern formal usage still shies away from certain constructions ending with a preposition, these are no longer absolutely prohibited. They are most likely to find acceptance when, as in the last example above, the preposition works in close concert with a verb: *hear of, believe in, interfere with*.

A **conjunction** introduces a clause and indicates its relation to some other part of the sentence.

> You had better correct the adrenal failure *before* you start thyroid
>   replacement.
> I suspected candidiasis *but* I was mistaken.

A clause introduced by *and, as, either, or, neither, nor* or *than* may be abbreviated by ellipsis to a phrase or even a single word.

> They gave him much more time than [they gave] me.
> Either the surgeon [will have to assume that responsibility] or
>   the anesthesiologist will have to assume that responsibility.

Correlative conjunctions (*either . . . or, neither . . . nor, not only . . . but also*) work in pairs. The clauses introduced by such a pair ought to be parallel in construction.

> *Either he fell or was pushed from a window sill.

RECAST:

$$\text{He} \begin{cases} \text{either} \quad \text{fell} \\ \text{or} \quad \text{was pushed} \end{cases} \text{from a window sill.}$$

OR:

$$\begin{cases} \text{Either} \quad \text{he fell} \\ \text{or} \quad \text{he was pushed} \end{cases} \text{from a window sill.}$$

In speech the conjunction *that* is often omitted after a verb denoting thinking or saying. This usage is acceptable in print when the meaning is clear.

The patient said ∧ he believed ∧ he had swallowed a coin.

Avoid the following colloquial or substandard constructions in formal writing.

*False negative or equivocal angiographic diagnoses occur frequently enough *so* certain pitfalls should be mentioned.
BETTER: frequently enough *that*
*He had been taking probenecid for so long he forgot why it was prescribed. BETTER: so long *that* he forgot

A **relative pronoun** operates like a conjunction by joining to its antecedent a relative clause of which it is a part. The relative pronouns are *who, whom, which* and *that*.

Not every patient *who* returned had taken the medicine *that* was prescribed.

A *restricting* or *essential relative clause* defines or distinguishes the antecedent of its relative pronoun. It is not set off by commas.

We prepared a list of the patients *who were lost to follow-up*. (The relative clause states an essential and distinguishing feature of the patients on the list.)

In speech the relative pronoun is often dropped from a restricting relative clause. This omission is acceptable in formal writing when the resulting construction is perfectly intelligible.

> The patient was asked repeatedly to bring in all the medicine
> he had been taking.

A *nonrestricting* or *nonessential relative clause* merely describes the antecedent of the relative pronoun. It can be omitted without changing the sense of the main clause, from which it is separated by a comma or commas.

> This girl had a similar rash four years ago, *for which she was treated with prednisone.*
> The patients in group D, *who received only placebo,* showed a higher rate of relapse.

The relative pronoun *that* introduces restricting clauses only. *Which* may introduce either kind of clause; the rule confining it to nonrestricting clauses is an invention of grammarians and editors, and does not accurately reflect good usage. *Which* is often preferable when the conjunction *that* appears in or near a restricting relative clause.

> It is apparent that the rats which Barbier studied were an inbred strain.

Moreover, after the demonstrative pronoun *that* the relative *that* is almost unthinkable.

> The only residue obtainable was that which adhered to the glass mouth of the receiver.

Finally, *which* is mandatory as the object of a preposition.

> Choose a syringe in which the plunger moves rather loosely.

Whom, nearly extinct in speech, is the expected form in writing when the pronoun is a direct or indirect object or the object of a preposition. The choice between *who* and *whom* in a relative clause depends on the role of the relative pronoun in its clause.

> Give this information to *whoever* [NOT *whomever*] needs it. (*Whoever* is the subject of the relative clause *whoever needs it,* not the indirect object of *give.*)
> He ordered a lipid profile on two patients *who* [NOT *whom*] he noticed had chloasma. (*Who* is the subject of the relative clause, not the object of *noticed.*)

VERBALS

A **verbal** is a form of a verb which can function as a noun or an adjective while retaining its power to take a complement.

An **infinitive** is a verbal which functions as a noun. The infinitive has voice (active or passive) and tense but differs from a *finite* verb in not having person or number.

> The only thing I could *do* was *remove* the entire lobe.
> I watched him *swallow* both tablets this morning.

An infinitive is the only complement possible for the verbs *can* (as in the example above), *must* and *ought*. The direct object of *let, permit* or *allow* may be an infinitive; the person or thing given permission is then the indirect object.

	IND. OBJ.	DIR. OBJ.	
Permit	the thyroid	to recover	its function.

The infinitive most often appears in an adjectival or adverbial phrase introduced by *to*.

> The time *to incise* and *drain* this lesion has not yet arrived.
> Maintain full dosage for at least one month *to prevent* relapse.
> *To judge* by his electrolytes, vomiting has not played a major role in his dehydration.

In the last example an adverbial phrase containing an infinitive modifies an entire sentence.

The infinitive is regularly introduced by *to* even when it functions as a pure noun.

> To digitalize may be the greater of two evils.

The expletive *it* often figures in infinitive constructions.

> *It* should be unnecessary to remind the reader that *it* may be impossible to identify advanced retinal disease until after cataract extraction.

Another common infinitive construction is an inversion such as the following.

That is easy for you to say. (*That* is not the subject of the sentence but the object of *say*. The subject is the infinitive.)

An infinitive may be modified by an adverb but never by an adjective.
A split infinitive is one which is separated from the introductory *to* by an
adverb or other word (*to already have, to seldom complain*). This construction was damned by traditional grammarians as a barbarism. Many
distinguished modern writers contrive to avoid the split infinitive without
substituting awkward or ambiguous constructions. Even those who find
nothing inherently objectionable in split infinitives must admit that they
are sometimes clumsy or misleading.

A **gerund** is also a verbal noun. It always ends in *-ing*.

Reducing the solute load may correct dehydration by *allowing*
physiologic retention of ingested water.

A gerund may be modified by an adjective only when it does not take
an object.

Remove the cap with a gentle tapping.
Remove the cap by tapping it gently.

The "subject" of a gerund is often indicated by a genitive.

What is the risk of this *child's* contracting polio?
They removed the batteries without the *patient's* knowing it.
I have no objection to *his* leaving.

The object of a gerund may also be shown by a genitive, usually formed
with *of*.

the suturing of the fascial sling OR suturing the fascial sling
the killing of Dr. Morgan OR killing Dr. Morgan

These constructions must be distinguished from the following kinds, in
which the genitive is not needed.

Continuous monitoring is the only way to prevent *it* [from] reaching a dangerous level.
We believed that the circumstances justified *him* [in] revealing that
information.
It is a pity to see *it* deteriorating for want of an application.

I do not approve of a *doctor* hitting a nurse with a stool.

In the first two examples prepositions have been dropped out by ellipsis (cf. *trouble sleeping, gone fishing*). In the third and fourth the *-ing* words are not gerunds but participles. (Participles are discussed immediately below.) However, not all authorities accept these interpretations. Some editors will insist upon genitives: *its* reaching, *his* revealing, *its* deteriorating, a *doctor's* hitting.

A **participle** is a verbal adjective. A *present* (or *active*) *participle* ends in *-ing*.

> The patient *having* a *sliding* hiatal hernia is more likely to experience gastroesophageal reflux.

A *past* (or *passive*) *participle* often but not always ends in *-ed*.

> A *fragmented* history is better than none.
> Bring in the lady with the *broken* thumb.

Note that a verb in the passive voice always consists of a passive participle and one or more auxiliary verbs.

> Results of liver function studies *had* not *been reported* when treatment *was started*.

A participle which is followed by its own complement or by an adverb or adverbial phrase or clause is best placed after its headword.

> These are the x-rays taken and developed at my office.

A *dangling participle* is one without a clearly perceived headword. Dangling participles are common and usually intelligible in speech. Certain kinds have the sanction of long and widespread use even in formal writing—for example, in an expression that introduces or modifies an entire clause or sentence, and in the case of a participle that has been fully transformed into a preposition.

> Strictly *speaking,* this is not a premalignant lesion but carcinoma in situ.
> *Continuing* the analogy of a balloon, the cessation of filling is succeeded at once by the initiation of emptying.
> This is either a recurrence or an exacerbation, *depending* on your viewpoint.

However, the majority of dangling participles are objectionable in formal writing. Even when their meaning is perfectly clear, which it often is not, they will be perceived by many readers as colloquial and vulgar.

> *Serum lipoproteins can be separated *using* flotation techniques and the ultracentrifuge.
> *Inserting* a coude catheter, the patient was relieved of 1350 ml of urine.

The first example is merely uncouth, but in the second there is a complete breakdown of communication. For the reader accustomed to using English correctly, the only interpretation possible is that the patient himself inserted the catheter.

The construction known as a *participial absolute* is acceptable, if somewhat stilted. It should not be mistaken for a dangling participle.

> The renal function *continuing* to deteriorate, she was transferred on Thursday to the County Hospital.

Faults with participles are discussed in detail in Chapter 11.

INTERJECTIONS

An **interjection** is a word expressing sudden or strong emotion. Ordinarily it is followed by an exclamation mark.

> Alas!
> Ouch!

Interjections are seldom appropriate in formal writing except when they occur in quotations.

PUNCTUATION

Written symbols other than letters and numbers are known generically as punctuation marks. The marks in common use in English include true punctuation—*full stops* (period, question mark, exclamation mark) and *half stops* (comma, semicolon, colon)—as well as *marks which sequester or separate* (dash, parentheses, brackets, quotation marks, virgule), *spelling marks* (apostrophe, hyphen) and *accents* (grave accent, acute accent, circumflex, tilde, cedilla, diaeresis, umlaut).

Oscar Wilde's assertion that he spent all morning putting in a comma, and all afternoon taking it out again, is not to be taken more seriously than any of his other witty effusions, but it underscores the critical role of punctuation in composition. It is no exaggeration to say that punctuation is as essential to written language as any part of speech or class of construction. As an example, consider the indispensable function of the period in signaling the reader that a sentence has ended. (How fervently teachers of grammar wish for so simple and direct a means of telling the writer when he has run out of sentence!)

Some practices concerning punctuation vary widely from publisher to publisher, while others are relatively fixed. Newspapers and other periodicals use less punctuation than books, and modern writers use less than writers of a hundred years ago. The guidelines given here, based on current formal usage, may require modification in accordance with the style manual of a particular publisher or editorial board.

A **period** (.) marks the end of a declarative or imperative sentence.

> Pyrimethamine is a folic acid antagonist.
> Hold your breath.

It is also used after a sentence fragment which stands alone and has the force of a full sentence.

> Can we find a single case of beriberi in the wards? No. Could Osler? Yes, on occasion.

A period is used after an initial or abbreviation.

Feb.	gyn.	St. Luke's Hosp.	t.i.d.	e.g.
Thurs.	E. R.	E. J. Bardon, M. D.	p.m.	etc.

Exceptions to this usage include omission of the period from abbreviations of metric units (*mg/kg*) and from initialisms and acronyms (*DNA, BUN, PEEP*). Some style manuals prohibit a period after abbreviations of nonmetric units (*ft*) and of Latin expressions (*ie*), after any abbreviation which preserves the last letter of the word (*Mr, Dr*), and after any abbreviation in a bibliographic entry (*Arch Derm, ed, Co, NJ*).

The period is typographically identical with the decimal point in Anglo-American usage, though in many other languages a comma serves as a decimal point.

An **ellipsis** (. . .) indicates that a statement is incomplete or unfinished.

> We had hoped to operate this morning, but with this fever . . .

This has little application to technical literature. The chief use of the ellipsis in medical writing is to indicate the omission of one or more words from a quoted text.

> "I swear . . . that . . . I will not provide unto any woman the means of procuring an abortion."

When an ellipsis ends a sentence some style manuals require a fourth dot.

A **question mark** (?) follows a direct question but not an indirect one.

> Where is my spleen?
> The patient asked where his spleen was.

The **exclamation mark** (!) follows a word or sentence expressing strong emotion. Except in direct quotations it is generally out of place in formal technical prose.

The **comma** (,) indicates a slighter pause in speech or a less complete suspension of the flow of ideas than a period. It is impossible to reduce to a few simple rules the patterns according to which formal usage inserts and omits commas. These must be learned from the example of good writing, not from newspapers, magazines and pharmaceutical package inserts. The following paragraphs indicate some applications of the comma that are well established and nearly universal.

When two independent clauses are intimately connected in meaning, they may need no more than a comma to separate them.

> In asystole cardiac contractions are not merely ineffectual, they cease.

This usage must not be confused with the clumsy error known as the *comma splice,* in which two sentences are incorrectly joined by a comma.

> *The patient denied illicit drug use, he claimed he had been poisoned.

A word, phrase or clause is separated from the rest of the sentence by commas in any of the following conditions.

1. When it is a substantive standing in loose apposition with a preceding substantive.

The fourth patient, a lifelong asthmatic, developed a supraven-
tricular arrhythmia.

BUT: His brother Edward also has a history of colonic polyps.
(*Edward* is in close apposition with *brother*.)

2. When it noticeably interrupts the flow of ideas.

This method, Stephenson reports, can be used safely even in con-
gestive heart failure.

3. When the sequence of words demands such separation for clarity.

Rapid atrial fibrillation requires, as a minimum, rate control with
digitalis.

When the BSP retention declines, other measures of hepatic function have usually returned to normal already.

If a hordeolum cannot be aborted, when it localizes it should
be incised.

In modern writing an introductory phrase or clause is not set off by a
comma unless it is truly parenthetical or unless the comma is needed to
prevent confusion. A comma always precedes and follows the phrase *that
is* (when it is used in the sense of *in other words*) and the Latin
abbreviations *i.e., e.g.,* and *viz.*

When a nonrestricting modifier (word, phrase or clause) follows its
headword, it must be set off by a comma.

There is a slight thoracic scoliosis, convex to the left.

He was later examined by the neurologist, who discovered nystagmus.

A clause introduced by *since, for* or *as* in the sense of *for the reason that*
is always nonrestricting and always requires a comma.

These reagents will have to be discarded, since they are obviously contaminated.

In each of the above applications, a comma must be placed both before
and after the separated element if that element is both preceded and followed by parts of the sentence.

Commas separate the members of a series.

He is allergic to dust, molds, pollens, animal dander and wool.
She denies intolerance to beans, cabbage, radishes, onions or
　　apples.

The commas in these examples serve as substitutes for *and* or *or*. Usage is divided concerning placement of a comma after the second-last member of the series, just before the conjunction (*animal dander, and wool; onions, or apples*). Though this last comma is usually superfluous, it is sanctioned by extensive use. A comma always stands before *etc.;* a second should follow it if it does not end the sentence. Commas may not be appropriate in a series of modifiers.

an ingenious new surgical technique
nonsuppurative nodular panniculitis

Commas are also used with dates, numerals and titles.

This patient first consulted me on April 18, 1966, because of weakness and weight loss.
The urine grew 100,000 colonies/cu mm.
R. E. Busby, M. D., will conduct the seminar.

The use of commas in bibliographic entries is too variable even for comment.
　　The cardinal rule for the use of the comma, a rule to which all others yield precedence, is that a comma should always be used when the meaning is thereby made more readily apparent, or when a likely miscue is thereby avoided. In case of doubt, insert a comma. If it is superfluous, the editor is sure to remove it.

The **semicolon** (;) indicates a slightly lesser degree of finality or separation than a period, but more than a comma. It usually stands between two independent clauses, with or without a conjunction. When no conjunction appears, the semicolon itself has a conjunctive force, often signifying *and therefore* or *but rather*.

The Bence Jones protein is usually not found on routine urinalysis;
　　it must be searched for with special tests.

The semicolon separates the members of a series when any of them is a phrase or clause containing one or more commas, or is very long or intricate.

Less common causes of intestinal obstruction are foreign bodies, including fecal concretions; tumors of the bowel or those pressing on it, such as mesenteric cysts; adhesions from acute or chronic peritonitis; masses of roundworms; and rectal stricture due to lymphogranuloma venereum.

The **colon** (:) stands before a sentence element that has been anticipated or introduced by what goes before the colon. The introductory passage may be either a full sentence or a shorter expression.

The deciduous teeth erupt in the following order: medial incisors, lateral incisors, cuspids, first molars and second molars.

A colon may also stand between clauses when the second elaborates, exemplifies or repeats the idea of the first.

The full irony of the situation became apparent only later: a simple blood pressure determination would have obviated the whole fiasco.

The substitution of a colon for forms of the verb *be,* common in journalism, is inappropriate in formal writing.

*At the radiologist's insistence, two doses of phenytoin were withheld on the morning of the examination. Result: the patient had another seizure in the afternoon.

The colon is used to express ratios, dilutions and times.

The rubella antibody titer was 1:10 initially but rose to 1:40 during convalescence.
She was pronounced dead at 3:40 a.m.

Parentheses () sequester material inserted in a sentence for illustration, definition, explanation or commentary when it disrupts the flow of ideas or does not blend smoothly into the syntax.

Such reactions have not been reported with Diamox (acetazolamide).
Even if the Epstein-Barr virus is the cause of classical infectious mononucleosis (and few can doubt that it is), testing for antibodies to it will not replace determination of heterophile titer, since heterophile antibodies appear much earlier.

A period is enclosed within parentheses only when the entire sentence is enclosed.

> The pulse increased initially. (That was exactly as expected.)
> BUT: The patient is presently receiving Lanoxin (digoxin).

Brackets [] enclose supplemental or explanatory material added to a quoted text.

> As Stroferson observes, "More extensive involvement [of the liver by metastatic tumor] may contraindicate surgery altogether."
> Parcher reported in 1961 that "Of twenty-seven deaths due to pulmonary embolism, twenty, or nearly three-quarters, were contributed [*sic*] by the attending physician to myocardial infarction."

In the second example, *sic* (Latin, *thus*) shows that the error appears in the original text.

Brackets also serve as parentheses within parentheses.

> Tarlton's method of treatment (continuous infusion of Geopen [carbenecillin] until culture reports become available) met with a slightly higher rate of success.

Since ordinary typewriters do not have brackets, these must usually be inserted by hand.

The **dash** (—) is used to separate parenthetical elements or to indicate an abrupt shift of thought.

> Prolonged administration of aminoglycoside— but only when clearly indicated—should prevent many of these recurrences.
> He also complains of postprandial epigastric distress—but that is nothing new.
> In grand mal, EEGs show a variety of electrical abnormalities, whereas in petit mal, findings are classical—consisting of diffuse, bilaterally synchronous spike and wave forms.
> Intravenous chlorpromazine may also be considered—unless there is a history of seizures.

There is hardly an instance in formal writing when a dash is preferable to some other mark of punctuation. Parentheses would be more appropriate in the first example above, and commas in the second and third. The last example would be improved if the dash were simply omitted.

Quotation marks (" ") enclose a direct quotation, that is, a verbatim repetition of words previously spoken or written.

> As Sir William Osler observed, "Errors in judgment must occur in the practice of an art which consists largely in balancing probabilities."
> The patient described his pain as a severe crushing sensation, "like somebody running a steam-roller over my chest."

When a quotation is a complete utterance, as in the first example above, it begins with a capital letter. When it is not a complete utterance, as in the second example, it does not begin with a capital letter unless it opens the sentence.

> "Jiggling spells" have sometimes been brought on by fatigue or alcohol ingestion.

Usage is divided concerning the placement of a comma before a quotation that begins within a sentence. In the first two examples above, the commas would be required by good usage even if the quotation marks were not used. After introductory expressions like *he said* or *such as,* the comma is usually though not always used with direct quotations.

> He said, "Pork makes me vomit."
> BUT: He said pork makes him vomit.

Quotation marks may be appropriate with a word or phrase of unorthodox or dubious connotation, especially when it was originally employed by someone other than the writer.

> Further investigation disclosed that the "parotid tumor" was in fact a quid of chewing tobacco.
> After receiving two more "adjustments" the patient developed urinary incontinence.

Quotation marks are best omitted after *so-called, allegedly* and similar modifiers.

> Her supposedly sedative medication kept her awake all night.

A quotation that must be enclosed within another is placed in single quotation marks.

> "We have reached a point," says Holtman, "at which further cries of 'Wolf!' will surely go unheeded."

When quotation marks must be combined with other marks of punctuation, the following conventions are observed in American printing.

1. With a period or a comma, the quotation marks always come after.
2. With a colon or a semicolon, the quotation marks always come before.
3. With a question mark or exclamation point, the quotation marks enclose the stop only when it is part of the question.

> Are we going to go on listening to his complaints of "elitism"?
> "What would you do," he asks, "if this patient were your wife?"
> And now they have the nerve to reproach us with "consumerism"!
> "For all I care," he announced, "you can just put me to sleep for good!"

The **virgule** (/) is used in writing fractions (*3/8*), compound units of measure (*mg/kg*) and blood pressure recordings (*136/92*). It is occasionally appropriate to separate words with a virgule (*albumin/globulin ratio*), but generally such usages as the following are to be avoided as informal.

> *Huebner postulates an infectious/toxic origin for this lesion.

And/or is slightly disreputable.

The **apostrophe** (') is used with *s* to form the genitive case of nouns, as discussed in Chapter 4.

> The patient's alarm was exceeded only by the physician's.

It is also used to form the possessive of certain pronouns (*one, someone, nobody*) and of *else,* but not the possessives *its, hers, theirs, ours.*

> One's perception of his own case is likely to differ greatly from someone else's perception of it.

The *s* is omitted after the apostrophe when it is not normally sounded in speech, as is the case with most plurals ending in *s.*

boys'   nurses'
BUT: men's   children's

Usage is divided in the case of a proper name ending in *s* or an *s* sound. The *s* is less often omitted after a monosyllabic name.

Wilms's BUT: Homans', Vleminckx'

The apostrophe with *s* may also be used to form the simple plural of a letter or symbol, but the use of *s* or *es* without an apostrophe is equally correct.

Map out the anesthetic zone with O's [OR Os] and the hypesthetic zone with X's [OR Xs].

In the 1920's [OR 1920s] the differential diagnosis of fever was twice as complex.

The use of the apostrophe to indicate the omission of one or more letters in a contracted form of speech has little application to technical exposition. Contractions are phonetic shortcuts which have not obtained much currency in written English. However, apostrophes in contracted proper names such as *D'Alessio* and *Prud'homme* should be carefully preserved.

The **hyphen** (-) is used when a word must be divided at the end of a line of writing or print. In printed material the dividing is of course done by the typographer. Divisions are made between syllables; a one-syllable word is therefore never divided. A single letter may not be cut off from the beginning or the end of a word (*i-buprofen, hyphem-a*). If a word is already hyphenated, the break should come at the hyphen. Other preferred sites are after a prefix or before a suffix. Letters which combine to form a new sound (*th, ch, ng, ow, ee*) must not be separated. Though these principles may seem simple and straightforward, they present some difficulties in practice. British and American views on syllabication diverge sharply.

The hyphen is also used to bind together two words in a compound expression. No element of typographic usage or "style" is subject to wider diversity. In many instances the hyphen may be used or omitted with equal correctness. Dictionaries and publishers' style manuals display extreme variation, and absolute consistency even within a single book or journal number is rare. The overriding principle stated earlier for the use of the comma applies also to the hyphen: a hyphen is always good form when its omission would leave a passage obscure, ambiguous or awkward.

In the following cases the hyphen may be considered mandatory, either because of nearly universal usage or because it is consistently needed for clarity. (Even on these points some style manuals disagree.)

In written numbers and fractions:

> Twenty-three patients died during the study period.
> The organization now includes 70-odd pediatricians [NOT 70 odd pediatricians] from the Bay Area.
> Nearly two-thirds of our series had experienced secondary failure on tolbutamide.

When a numeral and a unit are written together in a phrase used attributively:

> Take one tablet at 6-hourly intervals [NOT at 6 hourly intervals] with an 8-oz glass of water.
> For a 70-kg man, a standard 2.25-MHz transducer is more than adequate.
> A 28-day regimen is sound insurance against relapse.

With prefixes:

1. Before a word spelled with initial capital letter.

semi-Fowler, non-Polish
BUT: antiparkinsonian

2. Before a numeral, abbreviation or symbol.

pre-1920s, post-IVP, non- β

3. To separate identical vowels (but not consonants).

para-actinomycosis, anti-inflammatory, pre-existing, retro-orbital
BUT: posttraumatic, nonneural

4. To prevent confusion with another word.

Augmented sensitivity to re-sting [NOT resting] is presumptive evidence of allergy.

5. Usually with *by-* and *ex-*.

by-product, ex-husband

6. Nearly always with certain words (*all, full, half, near, self, large, small*) when they are used as prefixes.

self-discipline, near-starvation
NOTE THE DIFFERENCE: These dates are all inclusive.
These lists are all-inclusive.

With the suffixes -*less* and -*like* after *l:*

wall-less, wheel-like

In any phrase used attributively, when needed to clarify the relations among the words:
1. After a noun which retains its substantive role.

OBJECT OF PARTICIPLE: lumen-obliterating lesion, sternum-splitting incision
QUALIFYING ANOTHER WORD: hormone-dependent tumor, potassium-rich foods, gram-stained smears, maturity-onset diabetes

2. After an adjective, to indicate its headword clearly.

human-pathogenic fungi, close-grained fibers, first-order reaction
BUT: carpal tunnel syndrome

3. To join an adverb not ending in -*ly* to a participle or an adjective.

the so-called sodium pump, the deeper-lying ulnar nerve, broken-down erythrocytes, the last-named diagnosis, a much-needed solution, the now-quiet pneumonitis
BUT: a properly performed examination

4. Attributive phrase containing a connective.

less-than-effective measures, to-and-fro movement, left-to-right shunt, below-average values

5. Attributive phrase in which the hyphen itself acts as a connective.

crown-rump length, heart-lung machine, Stein-Leventhal syndrome

6. After an abbreviation or letter.

   PAS-positive specimen, B-mode sonography, T-wave changes,
      β-adrenergic blockade

The so-called hanging hyphen is correct when two or more hyphenated
compounds have the same second member.

   Diffuse theta- and delta-wave slowing may be seen in the many
      forms of metabolic encephalopathy.

This construction is generally acceptable also with nonhyphenated
compounds.

   Accurate diagnosis is a prerequisite for successful management of
      hypo- and hyperthyroid states.

In most of the examples of attributive phrases given above, the hyphen
is necessary for smooth, comfortable reading, and in some it is essential
to clarity. The use of the hyphen in attributive phrases is dying out in
newspaper practice and even in book publishing, to the detriment of
clarity and readability. In using a compound expression, especially in an
attributive way, carefully consider whether a hyphen would improve
intelligibility. If in doubt, use one. The reader will scarcely notice an
occasional superfluous hyphen, but he may sorely miss one incorrectly
omitted.

   Accent marks actually pertain to spelling rather than to punctuation.
Like letters they are phonetic symbols, but unlike them they cannot stand
alone; they can only modify the sounds of letters to which they are
apposed. English seldom uses accent marks other than the diaeresis (¨),
which indicates that the second of two vowels is pronounced separately,
as in *coöperate, diploë, oöphorectomy and reëxamine.* Even this mark is
now optional. With prefixes a hyphen is more common (*re-examine*) and
in other words all marks may be omitted (*oophorectomy, diploe*).
   The accent marks in common use in other languages include the grave
accent (`), the acute accent (´), the circumflex (ˆ), the tilde (˜), the
umlaut (typographically the same as the diaeresis) and the cedilla, which,
unlike the other marks, is placed under its letter (ç). Though there is a
growing trend in modern publishing to omit accent marks, they should
generally be preserved in foreign words that have not been completely
anglicized. As a rule a foreign word that is printed in italics (to be
discussed shortly) should receive its full complement of accents. Moreover, such borrowings as *exposé* and *resumé* may be misleading without

their accents. (Both *e*'s in the latter word have acute accents in French, but as a rule in American practice only the final *e* is accented.)

Foreign proper names should be given their accents, if possible: *Rinné, Ménière, Laënnec*. In German and Swedish the umlaut may be omitted and an *e* inserted after its vowel: *roentgenography, muellerian, Sjoegren. Munchausen* is correctly written without an umlaut. The name of the fictional character to whom the term *Munchausen syndrome* alludes is an anglicization of the German name, with two h's and an umlaut: *Münchhausen*.

CAPITALIZATION

The trade name of a drug, biological, reagent or device should be spelled with initial capital letter.

| Sudafed | Diodrast | Clinitest | Hyfrecator | Band-Aid |

Initialisms and acronyms should consist of capital letters unless convention dictates otherwise.

> BUN, FIGLU
> BUT: IMViC

Names of all taxonomic groups above species are written with initial capital letter.

The following should not be capitalized:

1. Anatomic terms: *oculomotor, profunda femoris, flexor digitorum profundus.*

2. Naturalized German common nouns: *anlage, gestalt.*

3. Words or phrases derived from proper names: *parkinsonism, wolffian, pasteurized, gram-negative.*

4. Abbreviations of Latin phrases, including *a.m., p.m., e.g., i.e.,* and pharmaceutical abbreviations (*b.i.d., p.r.n.*).

5. Letter designations of the waves of the jugular venous pulse (*a, c* and *v*), and *x-ray.*

ABBREVIATIONS

Follow a current medical dictionary or the publisher's style manual in choosing the proper form for an abbreviation, initialism, acronym or symbol. Some abbreviations are permissible in tables but not in text. Abbreviations for units of measure (*mg, cm*) are never pluralized, but initialisms and acronyms may be (*CBCs, REMs*). The choice between *a* and *an* before an abbreviation depends on the pronunciation of the abbreviation, not that of the full expression (*an SGOT level*). It is best to avoid beginning a sentence with an abbreviation.

An abbreviation that may be unfamiliar to the reader should not be used unless it has first been defined. The usual practice is to place the abbreviation in parentheses after the first mention of the term for which it stands.

> All patients had received donor blood tested for hepatitis H sur-
> face antigen (HB_sAg) by counterelectrophoresis (CEP). Subsequent
> testing of donor sera by solid-phase radioimmunoassay (RIA)
> revealed that three of the four hepatitis patients had received RIA-
> positive, CEP-negative blood.

Once an abbreviation has been explained it is customary to use it exclusively, without further reference to the full expression. This saves ink but requires much checking back by readers not endowed with photographic memories. Periodic repetition of the full expression would reinforce the informative value of the abbreviation. A still more commendable plan would be to avoid all but well-established abbreviations in formal writing. Perhaps only thus can the modern plague of initialisms and acronyms be forced to abate. (See McMillan R, Longmire RL: Crisis in oncology: acute vowel obstruction. *NEJM* 294:1288, 1976.)

Abbreviations that need not be expanded or explained include chemical formulas, abbreviations for standard units of measure (whether metric or not), those used in designations of time (*a.m.,* B.C., *Oct.*) and place (*Apt., Ave., N. Y.*), academic degrees, military ranks, bibliographic abbreviations and a few long-established medical abbreviations *(ECG, BUN)*. In a taxonomic name the genus may be abbreviated when both genus and species are given, provided that no misunderstanding can be foreseen (*P.* or *Ps. aeruginosa*). This usage cannot, however, be legitimately extended to other Latin phrases.

> erythema nodosum, NOT E. nodosum
> tinea cruris, NOT T. cruris

TYPOGRAPHY

Generally speaking the style, the size and the arrangement of type are the concerns of the editor and the printer. However, the writer is expected to show which words or passages, if any, he wants set in *italic type* by underlining them. Italics are useful chiefly to emphasize or distinguish.

In textbook writing and other highly organized and condensed prose, italicization of key words may be used in lieu of paragraph heads. In most bibliographic styles, book and journal titles appear in italics. **Boldface** and SMALL CAPITALS may also be used for emphasis in selected cases.

Italics are preferred for foreign words and phrases that have not been fully anglicized, but usage varies. If in doubt, consult a dictionary. A foreign word that can be found in neither a current unabridged dictionary nor a medical dictionary should probably be italicized. Italics are now seldom used for Latin phrases (in situ, sine qua non) or abbreviations (e.g., et al.).

The names of genera and species are italicized, but not those of higher taxonomic groups: *Proteus vulgaris,* Enterobacteraceae. Some style manuals require a genus name to be printed in roman letters with a lower case initial letter when it is used attributively: haemophilus meningitis. Terms derived from taxonomic names (shigellosis) and nonofficial designations for bacteria (pneumococcus) are always printed in lower case roman.

Use italics for emphasis very sparingly.

> *Infectious mononucleosis occurred in students *without* antibodies to the Epstein-Barr virus but not in students *with* antibodies.

The reasonably alert reader would perceive the distinction here without the help of typographic emphasis. Unnecessary italics create an undesirable air of tension and melodrama.

If you italicize part of a quotation (a practice that is not often justified) you must tell the reader so.

> "Any change in the distribution of pigment, *including uneven loss of pigment,* was considered an indication for excision." (Italics added.) OR: (Emphasis added.)

When a term that is normally italicized occurs in an italicized passage it is set in roman for contrast.

> If diagnosis is reasonably certain, proceed with treatment at once, but *do not overlook the possibility of concomitant* Ascaris *infestation.*

Any reputable printer of scientific literature has type for Greek letters and for chemical and mathematical symbols. These will have to be handwritten on the manuscript. Extensive usage permits substituting the name of a Greek letter for the letter itself: *chi-square, beta-hemolytic.*

When a Greek letter occurs at the beginning of a sentence, the first Roman letter is capitalized, but the Greek letter is not.

α -Adrenergic receptors . . . BUT: Alpha-adrenergic receptors . . .

NUMERALS

In technical writing a number below 10 is usually spelled out.

> Of nine patients observed for more than five years, only two required readmission.

In material of a uniformly literary or philosophical cast, numerals may be used only for figures over 99. The editor is the final arbiter.

All numbers, including those below 10, are printed as numerals in dates, times, ages, bibliographic entries, dosages, ratios, measurements or percents (when units or % are indicated), series of three or more and list headings.

> Death occurred at 2:40 p.m. on November 18, 1977.
> The patient was a 7-month-old Oriental female.
> *JAMA* 189:588, 1964.
> The initial dose was 5 mg intramuscularly.
> Serum albumin/globulin ratio was 1:1.3, creatinine 1.7 mg/dl and BSP retention 9%.
> All cultures (7 in nutrient agar, 7 in BPP and 2 in BHI) were incubated simultaneously.
> The goals of treatment, in order of priority, are 1. to relieve pain; 2. to restore adequate tissue perfusion; 3. to eliminate any known causative factors; and 4. to prevent disability.

In no case does American practice permit starting a sentence with a numeral. If a figure must start a sentence it should be written out. A unit of measurement following such a number is not abbreviated: *Twenty-one micrograms.* Ordinal numbers *first* through *ninth* are written in full, and those above *ninth* are written with the numeral followed by the last two letters of the word: *21st, 22nd, 23rd, 24th.* A fraction with a denominator below 10 may be written out: *three-fourths.* Fractions should generally be avoided or changed to decimals or percents.

Use Roman numerals only in accordance with modern conventions. They are appropriate as designations of clotting factors, cranial nerves and the standard limb leads of the ECG, and also with proper names (*Henry VIII, George D. Wheeler III*).

I hope it will not seem too violent an anticlimax if I assure the reader that there is hardly a rule in this chapter or the last which ought not sometimes to be violated for a good reason. The clear perception of such a reason, and the conviction that it justifies a departure from the usual practice, of course demand not only a theoretical knowledge of grammatical rules but also practical experience in applying them.

REFERENCES

A Manual of Style, ed 12. Chicago, University of Chicago Press, 1969.
Bernstein TM: *The Careful Writer.* New York, Atheneum, 1965.
Follett W: *Modern American Usage: A Guide.* New York, Hill and Wang, 1966.
Fowler HW: *A Dictionary of Modern English Usage,* ed. 2 (Gowers E, ed). Oxford, Oxford University Press, 1965.
Opdycke JB: *Harper's English Grammar* (Benedict S, ed). New York, Harper & Row, 1966.
Perrin PG: *Writer's Guide and Index to English,* ed 4. Glenview, Ill, Scott, Foresman & Company, 1965.

6

Accuracy

The need for accuracy in technical exposition is so basic and absolute that it naturally takes first place in any discussion of the principles of good medical writing. Accuracy means nothing more nor less than telling the truth, not merely when stating facts but also when reporting observations and deriving conclusions and principles from them. Since no one can tell the truth unless he first knows it, accuracy depends directly on the writer's grasp and command of his material.

The ideal of writing truthfully and correctly is founded on simple honesty, integrity and reverence for the truth, on respect for the reader, and on a clear awareness that the purpose of technical exposition is the dissemination of knowledge, not the attainment of glory, wealth or personal advancement. It is surely no coincidence that such perspicuous scientific writers as Darwin and Osler were known throughout their lives for their politeness and courtesy to all, as well as for their indifference to fame and wealth.

I have said that the purpose of technical writing is the dissemination of knowledge. A mistake is not knowledge, and neither is a lie. Inaccuracy in writing can always be traced either to an error, misconception or false conclusion of the writer's or to his deliberate failure to represent truthfully the content of his thought. It is outside my purpose to inquire into a writer's knowledge and experience or the authority on which he undertakes to inform and advise his peers. Still less can I address the question of his integrity, beyond stating the axiom that no academic credentials and no scientific distinction can excuse either carelessness or lack of candor in writing. Naturally all my remarks rest on the premise that the writer has something worthwhile to say.

Dishonesty in print consists less often in barefaced lying than in the author's arrogant assumption of authority. No one has the right to determine by himself what is a drug or procedure "of choice." (See Cole F: Method of choice. *JAMA* 237:2327, 1977.) No true scientist forces his observations or his conclusions into prominence by suppressing exceptions, variant data or divergent viewpoints. The candid and impartial investigator is immune to that selective amnesia that conveniently blots out of one's memory the contributions, and even the names, of forerunners and collaborators.

A writer must never let his fear of seeming irresolute, or deficient in his grasp of the subject, betray him into dogmatism or overstatement. Some matters are less clear than others, some principles less general, some exceptions less readily explained, some relationships not absolute. "There is no discredit," said Osler, "though there is at times much discomfort, in this everlasting *perhaps* with which we have to preface so much connected with the practice of our art."

One who writes with due frankness and sincerity does not engage in a game of make-believe with his readers. It is generally difficult and sometimes impossible to percuss the left cardiac border, to distinguish viral from mycoplasmal pneumonia, and to palpate the popliteal pulses. Since every physician knows these things, a medical writer who believes that he can impress his colleagues by pretending that he performs these feats himself with unvarying ease and accuracy is indeed naive. Equally disingenuous, though less liable to detection, is the trick of publishing impossible diagnostic criteria, costly "minimum workups" and treatment regimens, and similar idealistic or fanciful guidelines which far exceed the standards and routines according to which one conducts one's own daily practice.

The developing writer must struggle against the temptation to cover his lack of information with a rhetorical snow-job, to palm off muddy thinking under a veneer of smooth writing. The habit, once formed, is hard to break. A smooth presentation puts the reader off his guard, hiding abrupt and illogical transitions with the wax of empty words, and masking the cheapness of the material under a gloss of verbal varnish. The journalist relies on these techniques to conceal the superficiality and inadequacy of his information and the want of logic in his arguments; the novelist, to distract the reader from flaws and inconsistencies in plot and characterization. The conscientious technical writer, however, avoids these devices.

Among physicians writing for publication, accidental inaccuracy springs less often from factual error than from simple carelessness with the tools of expression. Writing demands far more attention to the relative weight and bearing of individual words than does speech. Nothing can be taken for granted. Nothing should be merely implied when it ought to be stated outright. Moreover, nothing should be implied that could not be stated outright.

If a writer were obliged to exhaust every ramification of every subject on which he touches, his paper or book would never end. Though some selection must take place at each stage in the development of a subject to keep the material within reasonable compass, this selection should be tempered by the realization that an omission may seem to the reader every bit as significant as an inclusion. The mention of a drug by brand name, for example, may be taken to mean that other brands are inferior. The mention of a single member of a class of drugs may suggest that it has significant advantages over the others.

It may be objected that readers who draw such conclusions are reading something into the material that is not there. That is exactly the point. A casual examination of the "Letters to the Editor" column of any medical journal will show how very frequently such misunderstandings occur. No subject occupies more space in such columns, with the possible exception of bickering over statistics. The writer must take his readers as he finds them and express himself on their terms as well as his own.

In performing his daily record-keeping chores the physician is assailed by numberless temptations to write fiction. I shall pass over in silence the mythical diagnoses sometimes entered on insurance claims, and the recording, after perfunctory examination, of reflexes elicited from a glass eye or a wooden leg. The well-established practice of reporting findings by negatives is a standing invitation to take liberties with the facts. "The thyroid gland is not palpated" could mean either that the gland cannot be felt or that no attempt was ever made to feel it. The formula, "The patient gave no history of . . ." implies, truly or falsely, that the patient was invited to give such a history.

Still more mendacious are formulas that convert negative statements into positive ones by gratuitous assumption of facts not known. Thus, having asked the patient whether he had any serious childhood diseases (rheumatic fever, scarlet fever, diphtheria, poliomyelitis), the physician may carelessly translate a negative answer into the positive assertion that the patient "had the usual childhood diseases."

Habits of juggling the truth in this cavalier fashion inevitably carry over into medical writing. The kind of medical fiction that most often gets into print is seen in the following statements, the like of which may be found in many textbooks.

*In placenta praevia there is no history of trauma.
*When an apical diastolic murmur is of the Austin Flint type, atrial fibrillation is absent.

Though these are what the logician calls universal negatives, they are not universally but only generally true. That is, they are not true in every particular case. They describe idealized versions of diseases, which (as every third-year medical student knows) are seldom found in captivity. Some women with placenta praevia do give a history of trauma; the truth behind the fiction is that this trauma did not cause the trouble. Some patients with Austin Flint murmurs do have atrial fibrillation. The truth is that the Austin Flint murmur, which arises from aortic valvular disease, must be distinguished from the diastolic murmur of mitral valvular disease, a condition more likely than aortic valvular disease to cause atrial fibrillation.

When the technical writer resorts to such generalizations he ought to make it perfectly clear that he is not stating a universal negative or affirmative. On the other hand, he must not hesitate to express himself absolutely and with conviction when justified by circumstances. *In general, may often, sometimes tends to* and similar mealy-mouthed phrases sound like hedging: they kick the legs out from under a straightforward statement of fact. Writing that is thickly strewn with such qualifications does not speak to the reader, it whimpers.

The factual content of a piece of writing may be roughly divided into what the author already knows from experience or training and what he needs to look up in a reference source. It is not in the latter kind of material that he is most apt to fall into error, but in what he thinks he already knows. A physician may go on for years, even decades, trusting in the correctness of a date, a percentage, a causal relationship, basing calculations or conclusions on it and teaching it to others, only to find at last that it is wrong.

The lesson to be learned, and learned well, is that every piece of factual material published, and especially quantitative data like dosages, dimensions and percentages, must be verified in at least one or two authoritative reference works. Once in print the most glaring error acquires a dignity, an almost inviolable sanctity. It may go on being repeated in other publications until the end of time, and may also prove an inexhaustible source of embarrassment to the author.

It should be unnecessary to advise the writer of a scientific paper to read all pertinent references and source material, making extracts and abstracts as needed, before he puts his first draft on paper. A competent clinical investigator will have done this homework before designing an experiment. Yet nothing could be more obvious than that many writers of scientific reports and reviews have never even seen some of the references which they cite in their bibliographies. How else can we explain the almost daily appearance of paper containing contradictions and misrepresentations of the very literature cited as source material and appealed to for corroboration? Careful reading of cited references not only adds to the writer's fund of knowledge and broadens his view of his subject but also gives him some notion of the relative merit or weight of his references. In addition, it prevents the jumbling of anecdotal reports with controlled studies and of case reports with review articles, and the still more pernicious blunder of including the same cases twice or more in a "series."

The reading must be done first. The typical writer is strongly disinclined to make any radical changes in his work once it begins to come into shape. Moreover, when the reading of references has been put off until after the first draft is down on paper, it is likely to be rushed through perfunctorily if not omitted altogether. Haste and carelessness in the review of pertinent literature may lead to faulty interpretation, particularly if the original material is obscure or ambiguous. In this way the ineptitude of one writer may bear bitter fruit through a succession of derivative papers.

LOGIC

The requirements of accuracy are not satisfied merely because all statements of fact are correctly and clearly worded. Conclusions and the steps by which they are arrived at must be no less sound and no less clearly set forth. Ignorance of the principles of reasoning, as embodied in the science of logic, is a severe handicap to the technical writer.

Classical logic dealt almost exclusively with deductive reasoning. In this purest form of reasoning, a general principle ("All guaiac-positive stool contains blood") is applied to a particular case ("This patient's stool is guaiac-positive") and a conclusion ("This patient's stool contains blood") is drawn. The conclusion is inherent in the premises and hence inescapable. Though such reasoning is essential to every valid diagnosis, as well as to many other mental chores performed in the trades, the arts and the professions, it has the disadvantage that it cannot generate new information; it can only restate the old. The "solution" 4 is predetermined by the statement of the "problem" 2 + 2. Finding this solution is an *analytic* process.

The great philosophic advance of the seventeenth century, spearheaded by Sir Francis Bacon and later augmented and refined by René Descartes, was the founding of what is called the scientific method, based upon experimentation and inductive reasoning. Modern science consists in grouping and organizing data so that general principles can be derived from them. The inductive process makes a leap from a group of individual and concrete facts to a general and abstract principle. The real world is composed solely of individuals; types and classes are an invention of the mind, and the statistician's crotchet, "Curve-smoothing approximates reality," is palpably absurd.

Induction is called a creative or *synthetic* act of the intellect because the conclusion is not inherent in the premises, and is not inescapable. Some of the data may be wrong, or the intermediate conclusions invalid, and yet the principle may be true for all that. If an induction is not subject to experimental proof it remains forever a theory. If, however, a crucial experiment can be devised, the induction is a hypothesis until it is proven, whereupon it becomes a principle, rule or law. If it is conclusively disproven it dies, or ought to do so. However, negative results in the usual sense would be more accurately designated nonresults: they should not be accorded the rank of facts, since failure to prove a hypothesis is not the same thing as disproving it.

Though pure logic does not recognize induction as reasoning, the scientific method uses deduction and induction together. For example, a typical investigation in medicine might include the observation and recording of qualitative or quantitative facts or relations under natural or experimental conditions, the induction of a general principle from observed data and its subsequent confirmation by further experiments, and the development and testing of techniques or methods. Deduction and induction are so intimately coordinated in modern scientific work that it is hard to find either in its pure state. The following examples are taken from *Pseudodoxia Epidemica* by the seventeenth-century English physician and naturalist Sir Thomas Browne.

In the first quotation the author uses a deductive argument to refute the myth that pleurisy occurs only on the left side:

> That *Pleurisies* are only on the left side, is a popular Tenent not only absurd but dangerous. From the misapprehension hereof, men omitting the opportunity of remedies, which otherwise they would not neglect. Chiefly occasioned by the Ignorance of *Anatomy* and the extent of the part affected; which in an exquisite *Pleurisie* is determined to be the skin or membrane which investeth the Ribs, for so it is defined, *Inflammatio membranae costas succingentis;* An Inflammation, either simple, consisting only of an hot and sanguineous affluxion; or else denominable from other humours, according to the predominancy of melancholy, flegm, or choler. The membrane thus inflamed, is properly called *Pleura;* from whence the disease hath its name; and this investeth not only one side, but overspreadeth the cavity of the chest, and affordeth a common coat unto the parts contained therein.
>
> Now therefore the *Pleura* being common unto both sides, it is not reasonable to confine the inflammation unto one, nor strictly to

determine it is alwaies in the side; but sometimes before and behind, that is, inclining to the Spine or Breast-bone; for thither this Coat extendeth; and therefore with equal propriety we may affirm, that ulcers of the lungs, or Apostems of the brain do happen only in the left side; or that Ruptures are confinable unto one side, whereas the Peritoneum or Rib of the Belly may be broke, or its perforations relaxed in either. (Browne T: *Pseudodoxia Epidemica* [1646] Fourth Book, Chapter III, Of Pleurisies.)

Apart from the final reduction to absurdity, Browne's argument is purely deductive. In the next quotation he presents experimental data to overthrow the popular delusion that the human body gains weight after death. The reader is expected to draw a conclusion from these data by induction.

That Men weigh heavier dead than alive, if experiment hath not failed us, we cannot reasonably grant. For though the trial hereof cannot so well be made on the body of Man, nor will the difference be sensible in the abate of scruples and dragms, yet can we not confirm the same in lesser Animals, from whence the inference is good; and the affirmative of *Pliny* saith, that it is true in all. For exactly weighing and strangling a *Chicken* in the Scales; upon an immediate ponderation, we could discover no sensible difference in weight; but suffering it to lie eight or ten hours, until it grew perfectly cold, it weighed most sensibly lighter; the like we attempted, and verified in *Mice,* and performed their trials in Scales, that would turn upon the eighth or tenth part of a grain. . . . (*ibid.,* Chapter VII, Concerning Weight.)

A point sometimes overlooked is that Bacon did not invent inductive reasoning. Abstracting general principles to unify and explain our experiences is just as natural a power of the human intellect as is deductive reasoning. If it were not, a whole army of philosophers would never have sufficed to create it. Whence came the universal axioms of the classical logician ("All men can see," "No horse can fly") if not from inductive acts of the intellect?

The very concepts of abnormality and disease are based on generalizations as to what is normal. The humoral theory of health and disease set forth in the Hippocratic Writings was but a misguided attempt to reduce observations to system and draw useful generalizations from them. At a different level of sophistication we have such popular "rules" as "A green Yule maketh a full churchyard" and "An apple a day keeps the doctor away."

What Bacon actually did was draw up rules according to which general conclusions might be validly drawn from individual data. His revolutionary methods, based on systematic observation, experimentation and the weighing of evidence, helped to dispel the empiricism and superstition that befogged primitive science, and to put an end to the slavish repetition and uncritical acceptance of vapid doctrines propounded by ancient philosophers.

The classical logicians evolved an elaborate machinery for the deduction of valid conclusions from various kinds of premises. However, they took no particular interest in the correctness of those premises. If, in the example given earlier, our major premise had been "All guaiac-positive stool contains diamonds," then the conclusion "This patient's stool contains diamonds" would be fully endorsed and ratified by the logician. By itself logic can no more ensure correct conclusions than can strict accuracy in the collection of data. All the same, logical principles must be followed in any deductive process if the conclusions are to have validity.

Violations of these principles have been dissected and classified as minutely as the principles themselves. An enumeration of recognized fallacies would take us far afield, but I may mention in passing two that are committed fairly often in medical reasoning. *Petitio principii,* or begging the question, occurs when the hypothesis or point to be demonstrated is taken for granted and included among the premises.

This fallacy is subject to many subtle variations, such as this example of a *circus vitiosus* spuriously attributed to Freud.

> FREUD: Everyone tends to deny motivations, experiences and behaviors that threaten his ego. The suppressed material continues to exert a subconscious influence but is not accessible to conscious introspection.
>
> SKEPTIC: Where is your proof? I deny categorically the presence of any subconscious forces in my psyche!
>
> FREUD: You deny them? There is your proof.

Another variation appears when the reasoner redefines his terms or shifts his frame of reference to deal with embarrassing exceptions to a preconceived "conclusion."

> TO BE PROVEN: Acupuncture cannot relieve symptoms of organic origin.
>
> FACT: Acupuncture relieves the symptoms of Ménière's syndrome.
>
> QUALIFICATION: Ménière's syndrome must not be of organic origin.

The most flagrant instance of begging the question, surprisingly common in medical argumentation, is the clumsy device whereby a hypothesis is railroaded through by sheer impudence. After listing several objections to his theory without even bothering to refute them, the writer returns to the charge by stating, with a total absence of logic and only the merest pretense at rhetoric, "*The fact remains* that rye bread cures viral nostalgia."

A second major fallacy commonly met with in medical reasoning is known as *post hoc ergo propter hoc,* the conclusion that one thing results from another because it comes after. This is a constant hazard in clinical investigation. The assumption that priority proves causality is implicit in the "therapeutic trial," and even double-blind crossover studies cannot entirely safeguard the researcher against it.

The rules of deductive reasoning and the means of detecting and avoiding common fallacies can be learned from any textbook of logic. Three excellent ones are listed among the references at the end of this chapter. Every medical researcher, and indeed every physician, should read Beveridge's *Art of Scientific Investigation* (see References), an admirably organized and beautifully written exposition of the scientific method as understood and applied in the modern era. The author, an experimental biologist specializing in infectious diseases, draws most of his examples from the work of the great nineteenth- and twentieth-century microbiologists, whose names, at least, will be familiar to every medical reader.

STATISTICS

The collection and handling of quantitative data are governed by an equally rigorous set of rules, the subject matter of the science of statistics. The researcher should always submit any quantitative findings to a professional statistician for analysis before publication. If the statistician is not a co-author, his name and credentials should be recorded separately. Some knowledge of statistical methods is required for the design of a valid experiment when quantitative results are to be gathered. Three reference works on statistics are listed at the end of this chapter.

The physician, no less than the investigator in the basic or pure sciences, needs to remember that the manipulation of statistics is not reasoning but only a highly formalized restatement of individual facts. The perilousness of statistical "thinking" unsupported by logic is evident in the familiar witticism correlating hospitalization and death: "Since most people die in the hospital, staying out of the hospital improves one's chances of survival."

For an excellent short review of common statistical fallacies, see Ludwig EG, Collette J: Some misuses of health statistics. *JAMA* 216: 493-499, 1971. Sisson JC et al: Clinical decision analysis. *JAMA* 236: 1259-1263, 1976, provide a brilliant analysis of the interaction of statistics and logic in medical decision-making.

BIAS

Nothing is so disheartening as the research project gone awry, the unforeseen hitch, the continuing accumulation of apparently meaningless data. Clinical subjects go to jail or commit suicide, a rack of serum samples vanishes or gets smashed on the laboratory floor. It is easy to fudge in the expected data, and easier still to believe later that those data support the expected conclusions. Despite occasional evidence that just such dark villainy occurs in medical research, the more common fault is an innocent and inadvertent forcing of data to fit preconceived conclusions. A subjective warp in one's perception of or attitude toward facts is known as bias.

Bias comprises many unconscious prejudices and states of mind which may condition one's view of scientific data and affect his manner of writing about them. The treacherous quality of bias is that it lurks beneath the surface and performs its dirty work without the knowledge or consent of its host. Moreover, its many forms cannot be analyzed and catalogued as neatly as the fallacies of deductive reasoning.

Certain prejudices and misconceptions are especially likely to bias the physician. Extensive experience as a clinical tactician is bad training for the scientist. Despite the broad scientific base of modern medicine, its practice is still largely empirical. The perpetual concentration of focus on the individual may sharpen one's deductive faculties while crippling his powers of abstraction. The pragmatic standards by which the physician reasons at the bedside, if carried over into his scientific thinking, will yield only misdirected, unscientific and barren inductions. One of the hazards of "pure" science is that of concocting groundless generalizations out of individual data. The practical scientist, on the other hand, runs the risk of concretizing abstractions in defiance of the most elementary common sense. In the next few paragraphs I shall describe some of the biases that are apt to afflict the clinician, without attempting an exhaustive catalog.

The *myth of the clinical entity,* according to which a disease is a real thing rather than an abstraction, comes into being because a concrete concept is easier and more comfortable to think and talk and write about. Though admittedly a kidney stone and an inflamed appendix are not abstractions, urolithiasis and appendicitis are. The distinction, being of little importance in practice, is scarcely observed.

The appeal of concretized concepts is shown by the fondness of both physicians and their patients for tangible evidence of disease or its absence (x-ray films, laboratory reports) and by the often-criticized practice of "treating" an abnormal x-ray finding or blood level in an apparently healthy person.

It is only in the mind that we can separate a disease from the organ or tissue that it affects. Though a tissue may be free of disease, no disease can exist independently of a tissue. Health itself is of course only another abstraction. Though the tie that binds together the components of a syndrome or "clinical picture" is purely intellectual, physicians tend to view any named group of signs or symptoms as an "entity" capable of subsisting in itself and of producing effects directly. Hence doubletalk like the following:

*Skull series is also indicated if the patient may be *a victim of* the battered child syndrome.
*Outdated tetracycline may cause Fanconi's syndrome, with *resultant* hypokalemia, proteinuria, glycosuria and aminoaciduria.

Perhaps because of the perennial fascination of the number three, a clinical triad is nearly certain to survive even when devoid of practical significance. Hutchinson's triad (interstitial keratitis, eighth-nerve deafness and Hutchinson's teeth) is a relatively uncommon combination of signs in congenital syphilis, and Charcot's triad (nystagmus, scanning speech and intention tremor) is an even rarer constellation in multiple sclerosis, except among patients with predominantly cerebellar involvement. Saint's triad is an almost certainly fortuitous association of cholelithiasis, colonic diverticulosis and hiatal hernia.

The *myth of the unitary cause* attributes a natural occurrence to a single cause acting alone. For instance, all the signs and symptoms of lobar pneumonia may be thought of as arising solely and directly from the action of *Diplococcus pneumoniae*. Complex functions may be considered linear, as when the severity of a case of pneumonia is thought of as varying along a one-dimensional axis, or the concentration of a substance in the blood as varying in response to a single determinant. This myth leads to the oversimplification of complex facts and phenomena and the lumping together of disparate facts having superficial similarities.

The *myth of primary disease* separates all states of ill-health into two broad classes. One comprises symptoms, signs, triads, syndromes, secondary conditions, complications and sequelae; the other, "primary," "essential," or "idiopathic" conditions. Such, for example, is the distinction between Raynaud's phenomenon and Raynaud's disease, between Cushing's syndrome and Cushing's disease. Though the basis for the division is that we do not know the causes of conditions in the second group, the myth has it that these conditions arise de novo, spontaneously, without any cause whatever.

The *myth of the malevolent pathogen* sees an essential difference between micro-organisms that do not cause human disease and those that do, the latter being hostile to mankind. Their toxins and other noxious products are viewed as offensive weapons, and their proliferation within a human host as a concerted attack against his well-being. This myth is fed by metaphors like *opportunism* and *virulence, resistance* and *host defenses.*

We sometimes speak of the patient's diagnosis as though this were synonymous with the patient's disease. Diagnosis is an act of the intellect, a feat of deductive reasoning. The doctor *makes* a diagnosis, which may be right or wrong, doubtful, probable or certain. The patient, however, does not *have* a diagnosis.

When we ask, "What is the diagnosis?" we do not, strictly speaking, mean "What is wrong with the patient?" The true sense of the question is, "What name has the doctor given to the disease?" or "Into what class has the doctor put the disease?" or both. From these two concepts of diagnosis come the labeling and pigeonholing myths.

The *labeling myth* says that the disease is the diagnosis and the diagnosis is the name given to the disease. "I am not so lost in lexicography," wrote Samuel Johnson in the Preface to his *Dictionary,* "as to forget that words are the daughters of earth, and that things are the sons of heaven." The scientist sometimes becomes so immersed in the organization and labeling of data that he forgets that the labels are distinct from the data, that they are signs which came after the things they represent and not before, and that they are in fact his own inventions.

>   *The fibula articulates with the tibia at both its upper and lower ends. Therefore superior and inferior talofibular joints are formed.

The second sentence, though conspicuously introduced by *therefore,* draws no conclusion or corollary from the data given by the first. It merely sticks on labels. Quite commonly a technical paper or book chapter which purports to convey detailed information turns out to be no more than an elaborate disquisition on nomenclature. A disease, for example, may be divided and subdivided into acute, subacute and chronic; chronic relapsing, chronic progressive and chronic benign; congenital, early acquired and tardive, etc., etc.

There is no denying the appeal to both patient and physician of a good resounding name for a disease, preferably with a little Greek in it. Diagnosis by description has given us such euphonious pieces of empty verbiage as *metropathia haemorrhagica* and *pityriasis rosea.* Indeed, the vast bulk of disease names, from *scarlet fever* and *tuberculosis* to *stiffman* and *restless legs syndromes,* are purely descriptive.

Some diagnostic terms achieve an unmerited popularity by being adopted as euphemisms. *Hypothyroidism* is more chic, or at least less damaging to self-esteem and public image, than *obesity.* In similar fashion *hypoglycemia* deputizes for *psychoneurosis, boredom* and *shiftlessness.* A *hyperkinetic child* may somehow be more tolerable than a *brat.* Equally appealing and equally unscientific are "wastebasket" diagnoses that refer to whole groups of vaguely related conditions: *cerebral palsy, hemorrhagic diathesis, nephrosis.* Though such terms may be of use in classifying diseases, the habit of applying them to individual patients after definitive evaluation smacks of diagnostic ineptitude and shoddy, uncritical thinking. (See Adelson L: Let's do away with CVA. *JAMA* 236:2390, 1976; Cole F: "Cardiac arrest." *JAMA* 237:2287, 1977.)

According to a highly plausible theory, the labeling of mental disorders is a societal reaction whereby the concept of disease is applied metaphorically to behavior that deviates in undesirable ways from the norm. (See Scheff TJ [ed]: *Labeling Madness.* Englewood Cliffs, NJ, Prentice-Hall, Inc, 1975.) Conversely, the psychiatrist and the clinical psychologist have labeled alcoholism and drug addiction as physical illnesses so as to remove their stigmata and enhance patients' responsiveness to treatment. Some observers believe that this practice actually reduces the efficacy of psychotherapy.

The *pigeonhole myth,* which compartmentalizes natural phenomena, arises from diagnosis by stereotype. According to this belief every case of illness ought to conform to some stereotype already fully defined by medical science. There are a finite number of possible "diseases" (that is, pigeonholes), and the condition of any person who is sick must fit into one or another of them.

Diagnosis, then, consists in putting each case into its pigeonhole. A disease that does not fit perfectly into any is "diagnosed" by being matched to the nearest available stereotype, on Sherlock Holmes' principle that when you have eliminated the impossible, whatever remains, however improbable, must be the truth. The physician who snickers over this ludicrous imitation of reasoning has perhaps failed to recognize the process by which he himself daily arrives at most of his diagnoses. Though a remarkably accurate method in the long run, it is also remarkably unscientific. Science establishes classes only after due consideration of the characteristics of individuals, and is in no hurry to broaden the limits of a class by adding members whose qualifications are in doubt.

The pigeonholing myth is responsible for the appearance in the medical literature of countless bizarre variants and *formes frustes* of known diseases. This myth is incredibly tenacious, considering that in practice it tends to refute itself. If a case that does not fit a stereotype is nevertheless matched with it, then either the criteria for that pigeonhole must be altered, or a new pigeonhole must be created. In the former case the "definition" of the pigeonhole is constantly changing, and in the latter the eventual outcome could be a number of pigeonholes equal to the number of patients. Either result destroys the utility of the pigeonholes.

An important corollary of the pigeonhole myth is the implicit belief that normalcy, too, is sharply defined—that is, that it has its own pigeonhole. This explains the physician's love of epithets that characterize normalcy: *afebrile, normotensive, euthyroid*. It is surely more rational to view health and disease as opposite ends of a continuum, and to hold that one disease blends by insensible gradations into another. The definition or stereotype of a disease does not reside in the disease itself, but, like its name, is a product of the mind.

EDITING AND PROOFREADING

In Chapter 3 I explained why a good editor is an indispensable advisor and assistant to the writer. Though the revisions suggested by an editor will almost invariably be found to improve the quality of your writing, the scope of those revisions is limited to the manner of presentation. No editor will correct your errors in dosage or catch wrong volume or page numbers in your bibliography. Moreover, unless the editor was a member of your research team, or made rounds with you when you were seeing the patients about whom you are writing, or is at your elbow as you write (all highly unlikely conditions) there is a danger that in making your words and sentences simpler, clearer and more attractive he may also make them false.

> *A hormone, or drug receptor, is that component of a target cell with which the pharmacologically active agent initially interacts.

The two commas, inserted by an editor who misunderstood the sentence, convert a simple statement into gibberish.

The following sentence appeared in the manuscript of a paper on industrial dermatoses.

> *Nickel containing stainless steel and other alloys rarely result in dermatitis, since the nickel is too firmly bound in the alloy to be freed by perspiration.

All that is wrong here is that the author omitted the hyphen that belongs between the first and second words. The editor, a better grammarian than metallurgist, took *nickel* to be the subject of the sentence, changed *result* to *results*, substituted a pronoun for *nickel* in the subordinate clause, and produced this piece of nonsense:

> *Nickel containing stainless steel and other alloys rarely results in dermatitis, since it is too firmly bound in the alloy to be freed by perspiration.

The story does not end here: both of these botched sentences reached print, and that was the fault of the writers, not of the editors. No matter how much editing your material has undergone, your name and not the editor's will appear under the title. You are fully and ultimately responsible for the truth, goodness and beauty of what is printed. Just as no reputable journal will publish edited material without letting the author review it, no competent editor will object to some dialog regarding the recasting of a sentenced which he has made more comely but perhaps less true.

Probably two-thirds of the so-called typographic errors that appear in print were in the copy submitted to the printer. Authors and editors find it less embarrassing to brand all mistakes in spelling and punctuation as typographic, blaming them on some nameless scapegoat with ink in his hair, than to admit any responsibility for such mistakes themselves. The professional printer, though, is not the half-witted drudge he is made out to be, and he could probably give your children's teachers some lessons in grammar, spelling and punctuation. But giving lessons is not his job, and whatever mistakes you send him he will set in type. Even if you do not believe the stories about fragments of tobacco turning up in the proofs as apostrophes, or flyspecks as periods, you may be certain that no printer will presume to amend your grammar or punctuation.

Though ostensibly the purpose of proofreading is to enable the author to catch genuine typographic errors before the work is printed, it also gives him a final opportunity to correct errors of his own making. It must be emphasized, however, that proofreading is not the occasion for a last general polishing of phraseology. If, like me, you receive your most brilliant inspirations after the copy has been sent to the printer, that is just too bad. Only the gravest reasons can justify extensive resetting of type, and in any event the author and not the publisher will probably have to pay for it.

The correction of proofs, a boring and nerve-wracking chore, discharges the author's final duty to his public. He may find it nearly impossible to review material for which familiarity has bred contempt with enough freshness of outlook to catch tiny spelling errors and misplaced decimal points. But regardless of the unpleasantness of the job, it is an integral and inescapable part of authorship, and the writing is not finished until the proofs have been reviewed and corrected.

ACCURACY: PRACTICAL GUIDELINES

1. Present information directly, candidly and fully.
2. Check facts, especially quantitative data, against reliable authorities.
3. Read all pertinent references before starting to write.
4. Get competent help with statistical design and analysis.
5. Subject all reasoning to a rigorous scrutiny to exclude logical and statistical fallacies and bias. •
6. Take nothing for granted; be explicit. Do not merely hint at what you mean, and take care not to hint at what you do not mean.
7. Review edited copy for possible deviations from your meaning.
8. Read proofs conscientiously and attentively.

REFERENCES

Barzun J, Graff HF: *The Modern Researcher*, rev ed. New York, Harcourt, Brace & World, 1970.

Beardsley MC: *Thinking Straight—Principles of Reasoning for Readers and Writers,* ed 3. Englewood Cliffs, NJ, Prentice-Hall, Inc, 1966.

Beveride WIB: *The Art of Scientific Investigation,* ed 3. New York, Random House (Vintage Books), 1957.

Bourke GJ, McGilvray J: *Interpretation and Uses of Medical Statistics.* Edinburgh, Blackwell Scientific Publications, 1969.

Burdette WJ, Gehan EA: *Planning and Analysis of Clinical Studies.* Springfield, Ill, Charles C Thomas, 1970.

Chase S: *Guides to Straight Thinking, with Thirteen Common Fallacies.* New York, Harper & Row, 1956.

Hill AB: *Principles of Medical Statistics,* ed 9. Oxford, Oxford University Press, 1971.

Huff D: *How to Lie with Statistics.* New York, WW Norton & Co, Inc, 1954.

Ingle DJ: *Is It Really So   A Guide to Clear Thinking*. Philadelphia, Westminster Press, 1976.

Pearson K: *The Grammar of Science*. London, JM Dent & Sons, Ltd, 1943.

7
Organization

One of the most conspicuous features of written material is its organization. We speak our thoughts with a freedom of association that would never be tolerated in print. Our sentences tumble out in nearly random order, even when, in narration, the sequence of our remarks is virtually dictated by the sequence of actual events. One sentence begets another by way of associations that are plain enough to us but not necessarily to our hearers.

A writer's orderly arrangement of his material does more than just conserve ink and time: it is itself a medium of communication. Words are not the tools of formal exposition but only its raw materials. The tools are the techniques by which the writer fits words together to show relations among ideas: definition, description, illustration, division, classification, comparison, contrast, analysis, narration, induction and deduction. The sequence of words, phrases, sentences and paragraphs on the printed page sets up a corresponding sequence of ideas in the reader's mind, thus expressing or emphasizing the temporal, causal and logical relationships among those ideas.

When you buy a lawnmower you expect to get a fully assembled machine, not 283 parts lying loose in a box. Having found your purchase in pieces, you would hardly be satisfied by the manufacturer's defense that "It's all there somewhere." You want something more than the sum of the parts, and you expect the seller to provide it. Similarly, more is expected of the writer than just getting all of his ideas down on paper. The responsibility for assembling those ideas, for making their interconnections perfectly plain by forging links of cause and effect, of part and whole, of proportion and variation, rests with the writer, not the reader.

117

Anyone who is unwilling to undertake a job of writing on those terms should have the decency not to undertake it at all. If he cannot get his own thoughts in order he ought not to presume to advise or instruct others. Publishing a farrago of undigested and disjointed fragments in the guise of a scientific paper is both an impertinence and a disservice to one's colleagues.

Before you set out to show the connections among your ideas in writing, you must outline them in meaningful order. The need for this preliminary blueprint of the material cannot be overemphasized. Even if brief, crude and tentative, an outline of some kind must be sketched out before writing begins. After all, if you are capable of writing the projected piece the outline already exists potentially in your head. You can spare yourself much time and effort by listing the main units of your thought in an appropriate order before you commit the first draft to paper. If you begin blindly you may end up repeatedly rewriting (or cutting and pasting) to adjust the overall structure of the piece. The work of revision should concern itself with the content, structure and sequence of sentences, not those of paragraphs, sections or chapters.

Effectively organized writing has a linear character: it moves the reader forward with each paragraph in a direction which the writer has determined in advance. By contrast, poorly organized writing tends to be circular. Plunging from one paragraph to the next without compass or rudder, the writer repeatedly brings his readers back to their point of embarkation. If his whole discourse were written out on one long strip of paper and the ends joined, he himself might be hard pressed to say just where the thread of thought starts or finishes. A writer who begins work with a faulty outline may find that he can maintain continuity only by relying heavily on rhetorical devices and by creating artificial bridges and imaginary connections in his material. This is the very antithesis of scientific exposition.

Some manuals of medical writing make too great an issue of the division of subject matter in a technical paper. Having read or skimmed thousands of such papers in the course of his professional education and career, every physician has a fairly accurate notion of the order in which the contents of a case report, an account of experimental findings, and a review of the literature are customarily presented. Surely no one who is qualified to write technical material needs to be told that the introduction comes at the beginning and the conclusion at the end, or that methods ought to be described before results are reported. Occasionally a technical presentation is badly marred by being hammered into a shape that does not suit it. It is essential, of course, to observe the regular format of the journal to which the paper is to be submitted, and to follow the editorial style manual if one is available.

As to the finer points of organization, the sequence in which ideas ought to be presented will usually be suggested by some other sequence: *temporal,* as in the narration of a case history; *causal* (from cause to effect), as in the report of a clinical trial, laboratory experiment or demonstration; *analytic* (from effect to cause), as in speculation or theorizing; or *logical,* as in argumentation. A temporal sequence seldom poses any problems, but the others can be extremely perplexing. Sometimes each of two paragraphs or blocks of material seems, for a different reason, to belong in front of the other. In such cases the deciding vote should be cast by the so-called *expository* order: from general to particular, and from known to unknown.

The grouping of material plays an integral role in organization. The simple and obvious maxim here is that like things belong together. Thus, whether you choose to discuss the advantages of a procedure before its disadvantages or after, you will naturally marshal these in two opposing groups instead of jumping back and forth from one side to the other.

The act of writing itself generates new ideas and new viewpoints, sometimes in great profusion, which may suggest radical changes in design. You must be prepared to alter your outline freely as your material develops. To make an outline perfectly flexible, put each heading on a separate file card and shuffle the deck until the sequence is right.

Since technical writing builds on a foundation of what the reader already knows, his comprehension and retention of new facts depends in great measure on how closely he associates and integrates them with his prior knowledge. A major function of organization in scientific exposition is to identify and reinforce such associations, reminding the reader of what he already knows and illustrating the bearing of that knowledge on what he is about to learn. Sometimes it is proper to deny an apparent association.

A cardinal rule in technical writing is to include only what is relevant. Though strict adherence to a well-drawn outline should keep the writer from rambling, the proper and logical dovetailing of his ideas demands also that he express them from a consistent viewpoint. The sections of a technical paper, unlike the movements of a symphony or the cantos of an epic poem, are expected to display a uniformity and evenness of tone. So strong is the tendency of the reader to look for unity and coherence in a mass of written matter that he will find it whether it is there or not. He tends to preserve a single mental setting or attitude toward what he is reading unless he is clearly told when the writer crosses the frontier between fact and hypothesis, between data and conclusions.

Lists, tables and charts require a particularly strict unity of form and content. A table may be thought of as a series of sentences stripped to the bone and inserted in a rigid framework whose physical configuration does the work of division and predication. The vital importance of consistency and parallelism in tables and other graphic displays of information is self-evident. Though these matters, like consistency in the typeface, type size and placement of headings, are principally the concerns of editor and typesetter, the author must accept ultimate responsibility for them, and carefully ascertain, in reading proofs, that typographic consistency has been preserved.

PARAGRAPH STRUCTURE

The effective writer never forgets that the order in which he places words and sentences before the reader is an integral part of the act of communication. His sentences unfold and succeed each other in a strictly logical cadence while seeming to flow forth spontaneously.

Each paragraph should deal with a single segment of material, these segments corresponding generally to the most particular headings in the outline. Often during the actual writing it turns out that a unit of subject matter cannot be elaborated within the bounds of a reasonably sized paragraph. Though there can be no absolute law as to the length of a paragraph, one that fills more than half a typewritten page will usually seem overlong to the reader. Just as the division of material into sentences lets the reader absorb one thought at a time, the grouping of sentences into paragraphs provides for a comfortable ebb and flow of attention. This ebb and flow is the key to paragraph structure.

The most primitive style of paragraph is just a list of facts. Their sequence is arbitrary and each stands in isolation, unattached to its neighbors by conjunctions or transitional words.

> The more severe and intractable forms of trigeminal neuralgia usually come on after middle age. The pain is often agonizing, and in a number of instances has driven the sufferer to suicide. In the form termed *tic douloureux*, convulsive twitchings of the facial muscles accompany the attacks of pain. Sometimes the pain comes on quite suddenly with great violence, and lasts only a minute or two. The attacks are apt to recur at very short intervals. Involvement of the maxillary division is often associated with migraine.

Usually a paragraph of technical exposition cannot be of so simple a structure as this. In the following example, taken from Darwin's *Origin of Species*, each sentence is tightly linked to the ones preceding and following, so that all together compose a tissue or strand of meaning whose coherence depends heavily on their structure and sequence:

The truth of the principle, that the greatest amount of life can be supported by great diversification of structure, is seen under many natural circumstances. In an extremely small area, especially if freely open to immigration, and where the contest between individual and individual must be severe, we always find great diversity in its inhabitants. For instance, I found that a piece of turf, three feet by four in size, which had been exposed for many years to exactly the same conditions, supported twenty species of plants, and these belonged to eighteen genera and to eight orders, which shows how much these plants differed from each other. So it is with the plants and insects on small and uniform islets; and so in small ponds of fresh water. Farmers find that they can raise most food by a rotation of plants belonging to the most different orders: nature follows what may be called a simultaneous rotation. Most of the animals and plants which live close round any small piece of ground, could live on it (supposing it not to be in any way peculiar in its nature), and may be said to be striving to the utmost to live there; but, it is seen, that where they come into the closest competition with each other, the advantages of diversification of structure, with the accompanying differences of habit and constitution, determine that the inhabitants, which thus jostle each other most closely, shall, as a general rule, belong to what we call different genera and orders. (Darwin C: *On the Origin of Species by Means of Natural Selection* [1859], Chapter IV, Natural Selection.)

We can perceive several forces at work in the evolution of such a paragraph from the mere list of facts that it might have been. First, the order of the sentences has been dictated by the needs of logic and exposition. Second, some thoughts have been expressed as simple sentences or independent clauses while others have been put into dependent clauses. Third, connective and transitional words and phrases have been inserted to show the relations among these sentences and clauses: conditionality and causality, concession and exception, correlation and disjunction.

Though the internal architecture of paragraphs is infinitely varied, we can identify a few basic structural features. The opening of a well-built paragraph starts a train of thought and generates an interest or curiosity which grows to intellectual suspense as the succeeding sentences develop the first idea. This curiosity is gratified at length by the closing sentence of the paragraph, which caps off the subject to the reader's satisfaction and relief.

This does not mean that the essential point of a paragraph ought to be kept submerged until the final sentence, like the solution of a murder mystery. Indeed, it is so much more natural to make a point first and adduce examples or proofs afterwards that when we find the reverse order we know that the rhetorician has been at work. In virtually every paragraph one sentence stands out as a statement of topic or theme, echoing the outline entry of which that paragraph is an elaboration. Normally this sentence is the most general one in the paragraph, the others providing examples, exceptions, proofs, deductions or details. It is chiefly to the position of this topic or theme sentence that we refer when we speak of paragraph structure.

A paragraph which comes straight to the point by beginning with its topic sentence, like the one just quoted from Darwin, may be called *natural,* and one which holds back the statement of its general point or thesis until the end may be called *inverted.* The nomenclature according to which these are styled respectively *deductive* and *inductive* runs the risk of confusion with the two kinds of reasoning discussed in the last chapter. (It will be noted that the examples of inductive and deductive reasoning quoted there from Sir Thomas Browne are both in what I have called natural order.) The central issue in paragraph structure is not the kind of reasoning set forth (if any) but the position of the thematic statement.

The inverted paragraph, a contrivance of the orator and the novelist, is ill suited to technical prose. The full bearing and weight of the particular facts imparted in a paragraph will be far more evident if a general statement about them has gone before. Two legitimate and useful devices in technical exposition must not be confused with paragraph inversion. One is restating the theme, or concisely recapitulating the salient points, at the end of the paragraph; this may be of particular value when the matter is intricate or abstruse. The other is announcing, at the end of one paragraph, the topic of the next.

> . . . Even suicide in depression is less the supreme punishment than the ultimate flight from reality. Punishment imposed by the depressed neurotic upon himself seldom suffices to erase psychological guilt. Indeed, his incapacity for imposing condign penalties on himself only adds to his frustration and guilt. In contrast, punishment imposed from without may lessen guilt by approximating divine retribution.
>
> A plausible demonstration of this fact is the observation that neurotic depression is often dissipated, temporarily or permanently, by the appearance of some external source of anxiety, grief or anger. . . .

The boundaries of a paragraph are far more flexible and arbitrary than those of a sentence. Indeed, in the last analysis the division of a text into paragraphs is just a typographic device for the convenience of the reader; such could certainly not be said of its division into sentences. Not all paragraphs, as printed, can be classified as natural or inverted. The following is an example of what has been called the *discursive* style.

> In regard to animals, much fewer experiments have been carefully tried than with plants. If our systematic arrangements can be trusted, that is if the genera of animals are as distinct from each other, as are the genera of plants, then we may infer that animals more widely separated in the scale of nature can be more easily crossed than in the case of plants; but the hybrids themselves are, I think, more sterile. I doubt whether any case of a perfectly fertile hybrid animal can be considered as thoroughly well authenticated. It should, however, be borne in mind that owing to few animals breeding freely under confinement, few experiments have been fairly tried: for instance, the canary-bird has been crossed with nine other finches, but as not one of these nine species breeds freely in confinement, we have no right to expect that the first crosses between them and the canary, or that their hybrids, should be perfectly fertile. Again, with respect to the fertility in successive generations of the more fertile hybrid animals, I hardly know of an instance in which two families of the same hybrid have been raised at the same time from different parents, so as to avoid the ill effects of close interbreeding. On the contrary, brothers and sisters have usually been crossed in each successive generation, in opposition to the constantly repeated admonition of every breeder. And in this case, it is not at all surprising that the inherent sterility in the hybrids should have gone on increasing. If we were to act thus, and pair brothers and sisters in the case of any pure animal, which from any cause had the least tendency to sterility, the breed would assuredly be lost in a very few generations. (Darwin C: *op. cit.*, Chapter VIII, Hybridism.)

A careful rereading of this selection will show that it actually comprises three rather sharply defined "paragraphs," each with its own topic sentence. Nearly every discursive paragraph will be found on examination to contain two or more paragraphs typographically welded together. There is nothing objectionable in this practice, though the modern writer is not advised to take Darwin as his model in the matter of paragraph length.

CONTINUITY

The coherence and continuity of writing depend on the structure and coordination of both sentences and paragraphs, but more particularly the former. "It is in the *relation* of sentences," said DeQuincey, "that the true life of composition resides. The mode of their *nexus*—the way in which one sentence is made to arise out of another, and to prepare the opening for a third—this is the great loom in which the textile process of the moving intellect reveals itself and prospers."

It is perfectly possible for two adjacent sentences to have no particular semantic connection. It is also possible for them to be so intimately associated in idea that no apparatus whatever is needed to show their relation. In most cases, however, the writer must expend at least a little effort on maintaining continuity between one sentence and the next. He would do well to keep in the back of his mind the old-time preacher's maxim: "Tell them what you're going to say, say it, and then tell them what you've said." (Unlike the preacher, the technical writer had better not spend equal time on each phase of his discourse.)

A reader should never have to stop and ask himself why this sentence follows that—whether it is meant to extend or elaborate on what went before, to draw a conclusion from it, or to introduce a new topic or point of view. He should never be in doubt whether the second sentence gives an example, a proof or an exception with respect to the first. Notice that in reading Darwin's paragraph on infertility in hybrids you never lose your bearings, or fail to see the links between the ideas.

With apologies to the shade of that estimable neurasthenic, I here present a recasting of his paragraph with all connective and directive words removed. It is, I think, a perfectly conclusive demonstration of the principle that juxtaposition is not exposition.

> In regard to animals few experiments have been tried. Our systematic arrangements may be trustworthy. The genera of animals may be distinct from each other. Some animals may be easily crossed. I think hybrids are sterile. I doubt whether any case of a fertile hybrid is authentic. Few animals breed freely under confinement. Few experiments have been fairly tried. The canary-bird has been crossed with nine other finches. None of these nine breeds freely in confinement. We should not expect first crosses between these nine species and the canary or their hybrids to be fertile. I know of no instance in which two families of the same hybrid have been raised at the same time from different parents. Brothers and sisters have been crossed in each successive generation. The inherent sterility in the hybrids increases. We might pair brothers and sisters in the case of a pure animal. The breed might be lost in a very few generations.

A transitional sentence serves as a coupling device to show how two paragraphs are related. Not every paragraph needs a transitional sentence, since not every one makes a transition. Moreover, establishing the connection need not use up a whole sentence. A single word (*next, accordingly*) or phrase (*by contrast, in exceptional cases*) inserted in the first sentence of a paragraph turns it into a transitional sentence. Conjunctions and adverbs can join paragraphs together as effectively as they can join clauses.

A good transitional sentence is both brief and pithy: it does its share of imparting information. A sentence that is purely transitional may interrupt continuity instead of preserving it, and so may a supposed transitional sentence that does not in fact carry the reader forward and across to a new vista.

> *This, however, is not by any means the full extent of the subject. Numerous other studies have shown that these organisms can withstand extreme drying.

The first sentence cannot truly be called transitional, since it gets us nowhere. All it does is drop a vague hint and leave us with a question. It might be objected that that question is answered by the second sentence; then why have the first one? The word *other* in the second sentence is all the connective apparatus needed here.

There can be no fixed rule for the position of a transitional sentence. It may stand at the end of one paragraph or the beginning of the next. When the transition is made at the opening of a paragraph laid out in natural order, the first sentence will normally combine topical and transitional functions. This is perhaps the commonest and most desirable arrangement. An equally suitable variation places the transitional sentence first, giving it a share of the topical statement, which is rounded off in the second.

> These endometrial changes that characterize the full estrous or menstrual cycle are not due wholly to the influence of estrogen. On the contrary, the culminating events that make the estrogen-primed endometrium suitable for pregnancy are directed by progesterone from the corpus luteum.

The idea is not, of course, to produce either topical or transitional sentences whose function is so evident that they stand out from all other sentences like uniformed policemen in the midst of a crowd; quite the reverse. The height of the tailor's art is hiding his seams, not drawing attention to them. Still, there is no merit in making a transition so subtly that the reader is unaware of it until it is long past.

Writing can never be too well organized, but it can labor under an excessive burden of organizational and transitional machinery. The writer with wide experience as a lecturer is especially apt to slip into this fault. If your ideas are well enough organized you should be able to steer your readers among them with a few deft touches of the pen—with a trim signpost at each crossroads, not a billboard at every step.

The magazine writer's trick of opening every paragraph with an eye-catching, attention-getting but wholly noncommittal sentence is cumbersome, artificial and amateurish. Such an overworking of the organizational apparatus serves only to conceal the absence of anything worth organizing. If the technical writer does not give his reader credit for a certain measure of intelligence and discernment, his connections and transitions may so far hypertrophy as to strangle and bury his meaning. It is a sad story when an apparatus erected to support something collapses under its own weight.

The judicious repetition or echoing of a word, phrase, sound or idea is a powerful organizing device, which can sometimes smooth transitions from sentence to sentence and from paragraph to paragraph so efficiently that no formal transitional words or sentences are needed. A contrast may be effectively pointed by the alternate repetition of two or more words or ideas.

The practice of calling any skin wound a laceration is open to some objections. The distinction between a *laceration* (literally, a *tear*) due to blunt trauma and an *incised wound* made by something sharp is more than academic. Lacerations occur principally in skin over bony prominences—the scalp, the supra-orbital ridges, the point of the chin, the knuckles, the elbows and the shins. Incised wounds may occur anywhere but are commonest on the hands and feet.

In a laceration, broken superficial vessels are often sealed off by the crushing nature of the injury, while deep vessels are unlikely to be injured at all. An incised wound may bleed copiously from cleanly severed skin capillaries and from punctured or slashed deeper vessels; hence there is greater risk of hematoma formation after wound closure.

The edges of a laceration are often so badly contused as to require debridement, but the wound is generally rectilinear and perpendicular to the surface. Though the edges of an incised wound are usually not crushed, it may be irregular in configuration, with complete avulsion of tissue, or may be so oblique that one edge is undermined and remains as a devitalized flap.

A laceration seldom contains foreign material except for grease or gravel; an incised wound is likely to contain a fragment of the cutting object, especially if it is broken glass or shredded metal.

As this example shows, the recurrence of a word several times throughout a piece of writing need not create an impression of repetitiousness or monotony. To try to induce variety by substituting a different synnonym for *laceration* and *incised wound* each time these terms occur would be to destroy the unity of the passage and perhaps scramble beyond recognition the contrast which is its main point.

It is sometimes hard to strike a mean between tedious repetition and obscure terseness. Some ideas merit repetition or restatement; others do not. In some cases it is better to echo a word or phrase exactly, in others just to paraphrase it—that is, to echo the idea.

SENTENCE STRUCTURE

We arrive now at the point where the theoretical yields to the practical; where, to borrow Thomas Edison's terminology, inspiration wanes and perspiration begins. The making of sentences, the very core and essence of composition, is a task of infinite complexity. Any attempt to reduce it to pattern or rule is foredoomed to failure. As in the case of the paragraph, however, I can offer a few observations for the guidance of the inexperienced writer in developing his own style.

The first requirement for the construction of a sentence is that it really be a sentence, and not a half sentence lacking subject or predicate, or a sentence and a half overflowing with words that belong somewhere else. The essential elements of a sentence, like the planks of a bridge, must all be present or they might as well all be absent. Moreover, there are no dark corners in a sentence where botched phrases may lie unnoticed, no rugs under which leftover words can be swept. Since each word and phrase in succession is fully exposed to the reader's eye, the selection and placement of each must receive a full measure of care and thought.

A second requirement is that there be no confusion about the syntactic relationships among the words, regardless of what rhetoric may dictate about their arrangement. The reference of every modifier, prepositional phrase and relative clause must be clear on first reading. These are points of syntax, not style, but the writer must keep them constantly in mind as he tries the various permutations of words and phrases suggested by stylistic considerations. Bad grammar is never good style.

A properly constructed sentence is not a gang of words standing around waiting for something to happen. It is not a mixture of combustible materials needing to be shaken or sparked before it ignites into meaning. It is not a random assemblage of parts, like the bits of colored glass in a child's kaleidoscope, needing to be turned many different ways before it yields up its full burden of ideas. A sentence is infinitely greater than the sum of its parts, because the order in which those parts are disposed is the key to the meaning they contain.

In the first chapter I spoke of the difference between a synthetic language like Latin, which depends heavily on inflection to denote changes in the sense and bearing of words, and an analytic or isolating language like English, in which word order is the principal syntactic device. In a synthetic language the speaker or writer can put his words in almost any order he pleases, because no matter where a word stands its inflectional ending shows its relation to the other words. Verbs cannot be confused with nouns, nor subjects with objects, nor adjectives modifying subjects with adjectives modifying objects, because each wears a distinctive label that tells the reader as much about the meaning of the whole sentence as the stem of the word tells him about the meaning of that word.

As an illustration of purely inflectional syntax, each of the following Latin sentences has a different meaning even though all contain the same words in the same order.

Nutrix aegro medicum invenit.	The nurse found the patient a doctor.
Nutrix aegrum medico invenit.	The nurse found the doctor a patient.
Nutrici aeger medicum invenit.	The patient found the nurse a a doctor.
Nutrici aegrum medicus invenit.	The doctor found the nurse a patient.
Nutricem aegro medicus invenit.	The doctor found the patient a nurse.
Nutricem aeger medico invenit.	The patient found the doctor a nurse.

Note that the differences among the English sentences reside solely in changes of word order, each word reappearing identical and unchanged in each sentence. Essential though word order is to the meanings of these English sentences, it is utterly devoid of significance in the Latin ones. Hence the concept of the sentence as a substitution frame (see Chapter I) can be applied only with reservations to Latin syntax.

The Latin poet, having no need of word order to convey his meaning, used it as a rhetorical and prosodic device, exploiting to the full the phonetics of his words and holding back anything he chose for the sake of surprise or suspense. In English the poet may sometimes indulge in inversions of normal order ("Bird thou never wert," "Lakes dark and deep sailed he across"), but there is a limit to the amount of bending and twisting that our language will stand before it flies to pieces. No one could get away with "Cain his firstborn Abel saw Adam slay." In these days when a taste for Latin poetry is no longer cultivated, the average reader boggles even at Samuel Butler's couplet,

> Diseases of their own accord,
> But cures come difficult and hard.

Indeed, so committed are we to our substitution-frame language that we occasionally misinterpret an inverted order in blind defiance of the few vestiges of inflection that remain to us, as did the orator who said, "Their hearts beat as one till death did *they* part."

The order of words in an English sentence may be considered from various points of view. *Grammatical* analysis identifies in each sentence a subject and a predicate and assigns positions to the other words and phrases which make their syntactic roles and references plainly evident. The *rhetorical* structure of a sentence refers to its theme, focus of attention or emphasis, and its continuity with adjacent sentences. The rhetorical "subject" or theme-word may be found in some obscure corner of the complement, and in closely knit writing may even lie outside the sentence.

> The liver is also capable of performing various oxidative processes. Vanillin, benzylamine and naphthalene are detoxicated there by this means.

The second sentence, like the first, is really saying something about the liver and oxidation, which are represented only by *there* and *by this means*.

Though the structure of the two short sentences in this example is satisfactory, ideally the grammatical subject and the rhetorical subject should be made to coincide. In a sentence as in a paragraph, the beginning and the end are the strong positions. The natural order puts the rhetorical subject first, while the so-called periodic sentence holds back the crucial idea or theme-word until the end. A child who says, "I have a tummyache" is not consciously constructing a circumlocution for the more direct and vigorous "My tummy aches." For him the rhetorical subject is *I*, and so he artlessly puts it first. Since writer and reader will often disagree as to what is the rhetorical subject of a sentence, any discussion of natural and periodic order must be slightly theoretical.

Putting a word or phrase first makes it the nucleus, frame or foundation on which the reader will erect his interpretation of the sentence as succeeding words unfold. The natural order, with the theme-word or idea at the front, is therefore particularly effective. This order is almost mandatory in a sentence which defines or characterizes something, or which must of necessity be rather long and complex.

If we think of every declarative sentence as the answer to a question, then a definition is the answer to a question beginning, "What is . . . ?"

> (What is beriberi?)
> Beriberi is a disease caused by deficiency of thiamine and mani-
> fested by peripheral neuritis, myocardial degeneration and
> edema.
> (What is rubella?)
> Rubella is a mild, highly communicable disease caused by a virus and
> characterized by a fever, catarrhal symptoms, lymphadenitis
> and a masculopapular rash.

When a matter of some intricacy must be dealt with in a sentence of some complexity, it is most natural to set down the central idea at the start, as a sort of sheet-anchor for the mind of both reader and writer—in effect fashioning the sentence as an answer to the question, "What is . . . ?" (The core of the main clause is shown in italics.)

> The *assumption* that plasma norepinephrine concentration is a quan-
> titative index of norepinephrine release and hence of sympathetic
> activity *is implicit* in the interpretation of plasma norepinephrine
> measurements, even though plasma norepinephrine concentration
> is a function of clearance from the plasma and the latter is the
> resultant not only of the release of norepinephrine but also of its
> reabsorption by axon terminals and its local metabolism.

When a sentence is not so complicated as this, and clarity and emphasis need no help from word order, a different principle comes into play. Nearly every sentence in medical exposition either asserts or negates the identity or relation of two concepts. The cardinal rule for constructing such a sentence is that the more difficult, abstract or unfamiliar concept should be put first, and the simpler and more concrete one held until last. Usually, but not always, this means progressing from the general to the particular.

Of all methods of treatment, past and present, proposed for the
management of diabetes mellitus, none has been found
superior to diet.

Most anemias developing during pregnancy are of the microcytic,
hypochromic type.

The commonest cause of superficial infections in man is *Staphy-
lococcus aureus.*

These are examples of the so-called periodic style, which begins a
sentence with the more general or abstract element and places the more
particular, concrete and specific one at the end. The final position
highlights an idea by concentrating upon it the focus of the reader's
intellect, a focus that has been sharpening and changing direction during
the reading of all the preceding words. A sentence of this pattern generates a delicate intellectual suspense, impelling the reader to the end in
search of an answer to the question or problem posed by the earlier
parts.

Long periodic sentences are apt to be confusing if not altogether
unintelligible, and even short ones put a strain on the reader's attention
if they come too thick and fast. For these reasons the periodic construction is best reserved for transitional sentences and short, epigrammatic
statements. A transitional sentence can be more closely tied to what has
gone before if it begins with some echo of the previous sentence or
paragraph.

A similar maximal transfer or reabsorptive capacity has been demonstrated for a number of other urinary solutes—phosphates,
amino acids and uric acid.

This finding has also been reported in a number of acute infectious
diseases and in various malignancies of the blood-forming
organs.

To start these sentences with the particular might have thrown the reader
off the track. Certainly it would have weakened the continuity of ideas.

The well-known line in King Henry IV, Part I, as Shakespeare originally wrote it, is "The better part of valor is discretion." Now that the
bloom of surprise has been taken off Falstaff's callow maxim by ten
generations of quoters, we generally find the statement recast in natural
order: "Discretion is the better part of valor," as though it were a
definition instead of a paradox. The original word order was periodic, a
construction particularly well suited to short, pithy sentences. An epi-
gram may occasionally be of value in technical exposition to underscore

or highlight an idea, particularly when that idea does not seem to belong in the topic sentence of the paragraph.

Though the inherent clarity and versatility of natural word order make it the workhorse of all expository writing, the unvarying use of the first position for the chief element in the sentence can generate a tiresome and monotonous rhythm in sustained writing. Some of this tedium can be relieved by the judicious use of introductory phrases and clauses. Generally it is poor composition to delay for long the appearance of the grammatical subject, but an introductory or transitional formula that is not too demanding or distracting may properly come first.

> It is hardly necessary to add that . . .
> Despite a strong preponderance of opinion in favor of the opposite view . . .
> BUT NOT:
> *As is true of most antiarrhythmic drugs, it is difficult to relate the clinical action of lidocaine to its electrophysiologic properties.

In the last sentence the grammatical subject (not the expletive *it* but the infinitive *to relate*) is held back too long. What is worse, we do not meet the rhetorical subject, *lidocaine*, until the sentence is nearly spent.

The reader must not take too seriously the technical distinction between natural and periodic order. As I have remarked already, it is sometimes impossible to decide which is the most important or the most specific component of a sentence. When two or more independent clauses are present, each will have its own orientation of parts. In a particularly long and complex sentence the main subject-predicate axis may be so buried in relative clauses and prepositional phrases that no one can say just where the core of its meaning begins or ends. (Try it with that one.)

Though the simple division into natural and periodic breaks down when we come to consider compound and complex sentences, one pattern may be preferable to others if it delivers its message more effectively and intelligibly. A sentence showing concession, contrast or causality should usually start with the simpler or more familiar concept or the shorter clause.

> INDEPENDENT CLAUSE FIRST:
> Hepatocellular necrosis is most unusual, though a few scattered parenchymal cells may exhibit early degenerative changes and may show evidence of active regeneration.
> Repeat challenge following recovery may be misleading, since several sensitivities may arise from reaction to a single drug.

DEPENDENT CLAUSE FIRST:

Though antibiotic treatment of meningitis has greatly reduced the incidence of complications, they are still of importance in those forms which tend to show a less uniformly favorable response to treatment.

Because the etiology is unknown, no method of treatment can be singled out as most rational or most likely to succeed, and none which does not worsen the patient's condition can be called entirely irrational.

In a conditional sentence the reverse arrangement typically, though not invariably, works best. Here the subordinate (*if*) clause should come first unless it is very short.

*Continued loss of insensible perspiration, sweat and urine will produce a net deficit characterized by loss of water in excess of salt loss if the patient refrains from drinking fluids and none have been administered parenterally.

BETTER: If the patient refrains from drinking fluids and none have been . . . etc.

BUT: Prognosis of burn healing at 24-48 hours usually proves accurate unless infection supervenes.

The order of grammatical elements in a sentence has hitherto received very little of our attention, since our examples have all been constructed on a straightforward subject-verb-complement model. Shifts from this pattern, besides injecting a pleasant variety into writing, have their practical uses. Because grammatical inversion is so striking a departure from what is expected, it can attract and focus the reader's attention as no mere juggling of rhetorical elements can.

OBJECT FIRST: All these hematologic complications our vigilance is powerless to prevent.

This we are about to discover.

PREDICATE ADJECTIVE FIRST, SUBJECT AFTER VERB: Few are the indications for such violent cathartics.

ADVERBIAL PHRASE FIRST, SUBJECT-PREDICATE AXIS PARTLY INVERTED: Only by repeated determinations of blood gases are we able to gauge objectively the effects of treatment.

INCORPORATED QUESTION: Whether these deficiencies can be corrected
is unknown.
What does seem certain is that current technology cannot cope
with its own ethical dilemmas.

Inversions of the first and last types make pleasing and natural transitional sentences.

One need not always resort to grammatical inversion to push a sentence element into the spotlight when conventional syntax would leave it
in the shadow. Discreet use of the passive voice, by making the receiver
of an action the grammatical subject, can give it a prominence that it
could not otherwise have without an awkward inversion. Of necessity this
device is used often in technical writing.

Pancreatic tissue and mucosal scrapings were minced, homo-
genized and washed three times with acid ethanol. The pooled
supernatant from these washings was adjusted to pH 7.5 with
1 N ammonium hydroxide and precipitated material was removed
by filtration.

Another way of varying sentence structure without doing violence to
grammar or forfeiting the reader's goodwill is using an expletive.

There are some cases, however, in which . . .
It may be impossible to state . . .

The term *expletive* has acquired a derogatory sense because it so often
denotes inert and meaningless words stuffed in among the needed ones.
Though an occasional introductory expletive is fine for variety, constructions like those above are best avoided in statements of major points,
since they clutter the valuable opening position of the sentence with
semantically feeble matter. Like the passive voice, expletive constructions
must be used with caution and restraint.

All of my remarks thus far have had to do with declarative sentences.
Imperative sentences are not of much use in technical writing except as
traffic signs ("See graph"). A sentence beginning "Remember that . . ."
is imperative in the strict grammatical sense but for practical purposes it
may be thought of as a simple assertion of whatever follows the conjunction. Naturally, a writer who is giving specific directions about a procedure or technique may find it awkward not to present his material as a
series of commands.

The medical writer seldom has occasion to write an exclamatory sentence, though now and then he may with propriety increase the impact of a statement by putting an exclamation mark after it.

Thus in the space of slightly more than four decades we have come full circle, and the substance once considered most useful for the prevention and treatment of these states is now implicated as their cause!

Questions are not entirely out of place, either. The rhetorical question, which does not expect an answer, may effectively demonstrate to the reader that a certain puzzle or predicament has no known solution.

When both public and private funds are exhausted, what resources remain?

A question can also be used to announce the topic of a paragraph.

What other processes are known to enter into the renal control of pH?

This device, so useful in signalling shifts of topic in a lecture (and in keeping the audience awake), may seem an eccentric mannerism in writing and must not be overworked.

It is surely apparent by now that no treatment of sentence structure can be perfectly objective or scientific. The distinction between abstract and concrete, general and particular, known and unknown varies from one observer to another. The surest guide to effective sentence structure is a taste formed by extensive and thoughtful reading and refined by experiment with one's own sentences in quest of the most intelligible, coherent and comfortable order in which to set forth words and ideas.

In this chapter I have discussed sentence structure mainly as a means of improving intelligibility and focusing attention. Many other stylistic considerations bear on the arrangement of words in sentences, among them exactness, parallelism of form, coordination and subordination, conciseness and auditory appeal. These and other determinants of sentence structure will occupy our attention throughout much of the rest of the book.

ORGANIZATION: PRACTICAL GUIDELINES

1. Outline your material carefully and fully before starting to write.
2. Include only what is relevant and arrange it in the order best suited to clear, logical and coherent exposition.

3. Plan the unfolding of material so as to link new information to the reader's prior knowledge.

4. Develop each item in your outline into a paragraph of text.

5. State the major point or theme of each paragraph at the start.

6. Connect paragraphs smoothly and unobtrusively by converting beginning or ending sentences or both to transitionals.

7. Construct sentences so that they interlock neatly and unfold the material in the sequence most readily grasped and assimilated.

8

Clarity

Writing is not really clear unless it conveys its intended message fully and correctly on the first reading. An aura of mystery may enhance the solemnity of religion, the majesty of government or the allure of woman, but it has nothing to contribute to technical writing. The chief ingredients of clarity are accuracy (saying what is true or correct), precision (saying it exactly) and intelligibility (saying it plainly).

Whereas you can judge the accuracy of your work even as you write it, you can seldom if ever form a perfectly trustworthy estimate of its clarity. It is the old story of the knowledge bias. The meaning of what you wrote is naturally plain enough to you because you were in possession of that meaning before it was ever embodied in words. Though the editor's first reading is the acid-test for clarity, you should be able to catch most of the obscurities and ambiguities in your own work by repeatedly and attentively reviewing it, gradually refining and sharpening its focus.

As soon as you have collected and arranged your material, write out your first draft as quickly and copiously as possible. Since accuracy and completeness are your first concerns here, you should waste no time on fine points of style. Leave wide margins to accommodate additions and corrections. If you use a typewriter, the lines should be double- and triple-spaced. When the right word eludes you, leave a blank. When a term seems inexact, rhymes unpleasantly with its neighbor, or needs eventual replacement for any other reason, put a ring around it. If you cannot decide between two synonyms, or eight, put them all down. All of these problems can be solved during revision.

Though perfect clarity is not to be expected until your work has been subjected to careful and repeated revision, it is a mistake to ignore completely the question of clarity in the first draft. Before we consider revision in detail, let us look at some guidelines for clear writing which should be followed from the start.

One way to characterize the style of a well-written technical paper is to say that it could readily be translated into another language. Ease of translation is a desirable trait in expository prose not only for the obvious reason that translation itself may be desirable, but because of what it says about the style of the original. The kind of writing that lends itself most freely to translation is that which always uses words in their literal senses and puts them together in a strictly functional way. By contrast, great fiction, poetry and drama, which are richly figurative and depend on cadence, verbal association and atmosphere to convey much of their message, practically defy translation.

Because we are talking about technical communication and not belles-lettres, we have good reasons for insisting upon literalness. It would be easy to translate "Our research into this question is still inconclusive" into any modern language, but how would you go about translating "This is Greek to me" into Greek? The literal meaning of a word is ordinarily the only one that is standard and precise enough to pass muster in technical writing. As soon as a writer's choice of words raises the suspicion that he is likely to use technical terms in a figurative, abstract or broadly inaccurate way instead of assigning to each of them its literal sense, he forefeits his credibility and, with it, his effectiveness as an expositor and communicator.

The English language is today a uniquely widespread medium, understood by more persons and used in commerce, science and government in more parts of the world than Latin ever was. In many countries where English is not the prevailing or native tongue (India, Japan, Scandinavia and much of Africa) it is nevertheless the customary language of medical publishing. Medical literature in English is read throughout virtually all of the civilized world.

By no means all native speakers of English are conversant with the nuances and vagaries of American English. Moreover, the work of an American medical writer will probably reach many non-native speakers of English, and many others with only a reading knowledge of the language. To such readers the literal meaning of a word, whether it is a technical term or not, is the first and perhaps the only meaning that will occur. A physician in Afghanistan, for example, may not even be able to find in his English-Persian dictionary any but the literal equivalents for such popular American words-of-all-work as *area, marked, involving* and *to deal with.*

Thus, the writer of medical English has a rather serious obligation to use words in as nearly as possible their dictionary or textbook meanings. This implies the avoidance not only of metaphorical expressions and enigmatic idioms (*last-ditch therapy, kid-glove treatment*) but also of colloquialisms (*elbow grease*), Americanisms (*flab*), medical argot (*edentulous and compensated*) and neologisms formed by analogy with any of these (*antihypertensive cocktail*).

Besides using words that can be understood by all his readers, the responsible writer always selects the word that most exactly expresses his thought, never settling for a humdrum formula (*embolic phenomena*) or a makeshift approximation (*cardiovascular aspects*). No amount of syntactic legerdemain can redeem a sentence whose words are not both accurate and precise. (Accuracy is hitting the target; precision is doing it with a rifle instead of a machine gun.) The conscientious writer rigorously avoids inexact clichés like the following.

> *There is *little agreement regarding the exact definition* of hyperkinesia.
> *The prognosis is *often less guarded* in viral pneumonitis.
> *A bone marrow aspiration was attempted but *a dry tap was obtained.*

Exactness in technical writing demands a close familiarity with the terminology of one's subject. Technical words must be not only correct but current. Anatomic and taxonomic nomenclatures are subject to periodic revision by quasi-official international groups. Generic drug names in this country are formulated or approved by the United States Adopted Names (USAN) Council, which occasionally simplifies a name or alters it to avoid confusion with others. Medical dictionaries do not ordinarily distinguish between terms in current use and their obsolete or outmoded predecessors. Thus, they may give equal space to *fallopian tube* and *uterine tube, diphenylhydantoin* and *phenytoin.*

There are, however, a number of medical publications that record current terminology in anatomy, microbiology and pharmacology. These, as well as the latest revisions of the American Medical Association's *Current Medical Information and Terminology* and *Current Procedural Terminology*, should be available in any medical library.

All journals now expect dimensions to be given in metric units. When a measurement has originally been made and recorded in English units, it should be so written, with the metric equivalent immediately following in parentheses.

> In 1961 the patient was 5 ft, 4 in (162.5 cm) tall and weighed 188 lb (85.5 kg).

It should be unnecessary to counsel the scientific writer against carrying out a metric conversion further than is warranted by the number of significant figures in the original measurement.

> *A truck driver reported blacking out suddenly after consuming two or three quarts (1.892-2.838 1) of home-brew.

Since apothecary measure (drams, grains) is now regarded as obsolete, dosages should be recorded in metric units, without apothecary equivalents.

There was once a paving contractor who said that he liked children in the abstract but not the concrete. A similar sentiment perhaps motivates the writer who tells us that febrile convulsions are more likely to occur "in the pediatric age group" instead of "in children." A weakness for abstractions is a common failing among technical writers. Setting out to record specific facts, observations, theories and conclusions, they produce only an amorphous blur of words that cannot be pulled into focus by any effort of the reader's intellect.

Some writers cannot bring their ideas down to the concrete, specific, sharply defined level expected in scientific communication because they cannot or will not come to terms with reality. It is far less trouble to think, talk and write about *resources, involvement* and *response* than to distinguish and identify all the things for which these abstractions can be made to stand.

At times, of course, metaphysical concepts and abstract ideas must be discussed even in medical writing. But if we allow ourselves to call enzymes, blood pressure readings and technical errors in the performance of inguinal herniorrhaphy all by the same abstract or philosophic term just as the mood strikes us, we rob that term of whatever specificity and definition it has in its proper sphere.

The practice of using general terms to introduce a deliberate vagueness into a statement cannot be too strongly condemned.

> *As with any new drug given over prolonged periods [how long?] laboratory parameters [which ones?] should be observed [how?] at regular intervals [what intervals?].

Achieving concreteness in writing demands more than just avoiding words that are too general, abstract or variegated in meaning. You must keep your mind as well as the reader's on specific and concrete things by dealing, whenever possible, with individual cases, facts or phenomena instead of classes and groups, especially groups that are held together by some purely abstract or intellectual bond. Thus, if you want to say something about long-term prophylaxis against bacterial infection in asthma, emphysema, bronchiectasis and chronic pulmonary congestion due to heart failure, you ought to name those conditions and not be content with a vague generic catch-phrase such as "chronic conditions of the lungs."

Beware of the collective plural. Not only is it abstract, but it leads to grammatical absurdities.

*Patients with tonsillar carcinoma may reach inoperability before they are aware that there is an abnormal mass in *their throat.*

If the individuals making up a group are too numerous to be listed, clarify your meaning by giving one or more well-chosen examples. You may find it advisable also to explicitly exclude things that do not belong to the group, particularly when the reader might otherwiser be expected to include them.

In the last chapter I stressed the importance to the writer of an outline of his material. An outline may sometimes be of great service to the reader also. The commendable practice of starting each chapter or section of a texbook with an outline or *précis,* formerly widespread and still in vogue in some countries, is regrettably almost unknown nowadays in American publishing.

Unlike fiction-writing, where subtlety and understatement are virtues, scientific writing demands explicitness. The medical writer dares take nothing for granted. If he wants to impart a fact or an idea he must state it fully, and not be content to drop a few hints, or give only disjointed facts and let the reader sift and interpret them. Explicitness in writing requires an eye for the significant, relevant, graphic detail, and the knack of incorporating it smoothly and logically into the presentation.

Many a paper fails to get its major points across to the general reader because it plunges without preamble into a subject with which he is only slightly familiar. Carefully consider whether a concise introductory section providing a few definitions or a little history would help the reader to grasp the material more readily. A common shortcoming of books with a dozen or more co-authors is that nobody lays the groundwork for a thorough understanding of the subject by stating or reviewing its basic principles or premises. This is of course an editorial rather than an auctorial responsibility.

Writing without emphasis is like music without crescendos. Even when not positively boring, it fails again and again to make its points. The simplest means of moving a word or idea into the spotlight is putting it in a conspicuous position. I discussed this subject in detail in the last chapter. Repetition, also discussed there as an aid in organizing and unifying, is a powerful tool for achieving emphasis. The advertiser shows his awareness of this when he intones the name of his product four or five times amid a blitzkrieg of doubletalk, unfinished sentences and innuendoes. Though repetition is presently in disrepute among educators, it remains immeasurably superior to any other method of impressing a piece of abstract information on the mind.

Instead of reinforcing a thought by restatement or paraphrase, the writer may choose to give it prominence by one of the following techniques:

EXAMPLE: Compulsive behavior represents a sort of penance done to reduce anxiety. Characteristically such behavior is repetitive and stereotyped. For instance, the patient may feel the need to touch every picket in a fence, or perhaps every fourth picket; to count or repeat certain words or numbers whenever a certain occasion arises; to perform a ritualistic washing of the hands or of some other part of the body to a degree far beyond the demands of cleanliness.

COMPARISON OR ANALOGY: The swollen, reddened and slightly macerated eponychium of moniliasis, with its tendency to separate from the root of the nail, has been likened to an old-fashioned bedroll lying across the foot of the bed.

A SHORT OR EPIGRAMMATIC SENTENCE: Diarrhea, with or without vomiting, militates against the diagnosis of influenza. Let us not be drawn into the error of the laity enshrined in the misnomer "intestinal flu." Influenza spares the gut.

A MNEMONIC: Since it is a flexor and supinator of the forearm, it may be remembered that the (right) biceps puts in the corkscrew and draws out the cork.

A VIVID OR MEMORABLE EXPRESSION: It may at times be nearly impossible to find the retroprostatic space of Proust, which has been so aptly described as lying "between the wind and the water."

HUMOR OR HYPERBOLE: The patient with a lacerated spleen or liver may exsanguinate into his peritoneal cavity while the surgical team is busy clamping and ligating capillaries in his dermis.

Even in your first draft you should pay close heed to the principles of grammar. Most of the sense-blurring faults of syntax to be discussed in

Chapter 11 could be avoided by the observance of a few basic principles. The principles are simple; their observance is not.

1. No matter how long and intricate the sentence, its subject-predicate axis determines the orientation and interrelation of all its other parts. The writer who observes this rule in every sentence he writes will never be guilty of creating dangling modifiers and orphan relative clauses.

2. Modifying words and phrases must be kept close to what they modify and away from what they do not modify. It is usually easy to keep adjectives with their headwords, but adverbs and prepositional phrases often wander far from home.

3. Though the path from the first word of a sentence to the last need not be straight, it must not fork, or leave the reader hanging on the brink of a chasm with no bridge in sight.

4. Clarity requires the skillful use of cues and signals, the proper and adequate placement of commas and hyphens, and the scrupulous avoidance of certain troublesome constructions to be considered in detail in Part III.

REVISION

When you have produced a first draft that is as accurate, as well-organized and as clear as you can make it, your work has just begun. Ideally there should be one rereading for accuracy, with careful checking of references and all numerical data; another for completeness and organization; at least one for clarity and conciseness; and several for readability, which will be discussed in the next chapter.

Revision can serve another important function that is often overlooked. In the heat of composition it is impossible to judge exactly how much or how little the reader needs to be told to grasp an idea. Revision gives the writer the chance to prune passages that overstate, overorganize or overclarify. Nothing in a draft should be considered fixed and unalterable. No matter how nicely turned a sentence, if it is inaccurate or superfluous it must go. Preserving felicitous deadwood at the expense of accuracy, conciseness or continuity is like sacrificing a life to save a limb.

Revision is most effectively performed in the course of a thoughtful and attentive rereading of the entire piece. Rough spot-revision may seriously weaken the fabric of a paragraph by bringing in an awkward repetition or making the text contradict itself. Sentences should fit together like the wheels and pinions of a clock, their sequence and relations subject to an all-pervading law of order and continuity. Seldom is it possible to change a sentence significantly without touching the rest of the paragraph.

Sometimes revision proves a grueling task. It may seem harder to patch up a bad first draft than it would be to tear it up and start afresh. Repeated rereading of the same material lulls the writer into inattention, so that flaws may escape his notice again and again. (That is why revision for accuracy should come first.) The distinction between revision and rewriting is purely mechanical: as long as you cross out words in a draft or insert others, you are revising, but when you copy the revised material on a fresh sheet of paper you are rewriting. By "revision" we usually mean both procedures. The decision to rewrite a page instead of just changing, deleting or adding words usually depends on the extent to which the draft has already been scribbled up and its margins filled with additions. Many great writers have been prolific rewriters, going through ten, twenty or more drafts of each book.

Intense and prolonged efforts at revision can induce a sort of cerebral writer's cramp. Prose that has been labored over too earnestly becomes as dry as overworked clay, as brittle as hammered brass. Instead of getting smoother and clearer it grows ever more tangled and obscure. Lay it aside. Only the rash and inexperienced writer believes that he can put the finishing touches in the evening to a piece of work that he has just begun that morning. "Easy writing," observed Sheridan in the eighteenth century, "is cursed hard reading."

Horace, having reminded us in his *Ars Poetica* that even good Homer nodded now and then, goes on to recommend that every piece of writing be kept back until the ninth year. If this is scarcely practical advice to the writer of a medical paper, it at least suggests the importance of his putting his work aside for a few days and coming back to it with a fresh outlook, to see whether it still makes sense to him. There is no piece so well organized and so well written that it cannot be improved by one more review. Even in the final revision, polishing of phraseology is not the sole concern. Some major reshuffling of paragraphs may be undertaken in the last stages of composition even by the best authors. (I am tempted to say *especially* by the best authors.)

There are four kinds of obscurity for which the writer should be on the watch during revision. The first and commonest is the slight rough place, the transient jamming of syntactic gears, with a temporary lapse of intelligibility. "How's that again?" the reader asks himself, reads it over, understands and moves on. The meaning is there but the writer has done the reader the discourtesy of making him dig for it.

The second kind of obscurity is ambiguity, which leaves the reader hanging undecided between two or more possible interpretations. More common is the construction which the reader misunderstands without even suspecting that another interpretation is possible. Finally there is the passage that makes no sense at all. This usually has to be caught and amended by the editor, since it makes perfect sense to the author.

It is often proposed as a defense of an obscure statement that the context makes the meaning clear. This is a feeble and ridiculous argument. The context may supply a word or phrase that is left out, but it can scarcely be relied on to correct a wrong word or phrase. Moreover, quoting out of context is a fine art, in which writers of review articles and textbooks display almost as much adeptness as lawyers and politicians. The "context" in which a phrase or sentence appears is not essentially different from the phrase or sentence itself. The passage under scrutiny is itself a part of the context of what precedes it and what follows it. Unless the whole is coherent and of uniform clarity, some part needs revision.

CONCISENESS

Since the essence of science is economy of thought, it is only fitting that scientific writing should be economical as well. If a technical writer dared rest content with a rambling and diffuse style, a dictating machine would suit his purpose as well as a pen. Indeed, unedited material often seems as prolix and disjointed as impromptu speech. With each revision its compass ought to shrink slightly, just as with each stroke of the plane a board becomes smoother by losing a little more material.

In the first draft conciseness is not necessarily desirable. Too strong an effort to concentrate your words at that early stage will only cramp your freedom of expression and cripple your creative faculty. When a painter starts with too small a canvas his work turns out tight and fussy. A writer cannot effectively edit his work for conciseness until he has learned not to be too terse in his first draft.

It has been said that a well-made sentence is the shortest distance between a capital letter and a period. The writer's thrift yields double gains to the reader, for succinctness enhances both clarity and appeal. Revision for conciseness includes two related processes: the removal of unneeded words, and the replacement of long words with short ones. It is amazing how much the readability of a passage can be improved by the removal of all words of three or more syllables for which suitable shorter ones can be substituted. Often it will be found that the longer word is merely a pedantic or grandiose variant of the shorter (*methodology* for *methods, musculature* for *muscles*). Of course, the substitution must leave the meaning intact. A *test* is not necessarily the same thing as an *analysis,* nor is *strength* exactly synonymous with *potency.* For many technical terms there simply are no shorter substitutes. Do not try to achieve brevity by using, in formal writing, such informal abridgements as *lab* or *'scope.*

The repellent habit of cluttering one's speech and writing with long words betrays the humbug and the charlatan. By contrast, the habitual choice of shorter words is one of the hallmarks of the forthright and unaffected speaker and writer. Our last excerpt from *The Origin of Species* contains scarcely a word over two syllables for which a shorter one could have been substituted.

> The causes which check the natural tendency of each species to increase in number are most obscure. Look at the most vigorous species: by as much as it swarms in numbers, by so much will its tendency to increase be still further increased. We know not exactly what the checks are in even one single instance. Nor will this surprise any one who reflects how ignorant we are on this head, even in regard to mankind, so incomparably better known than any other animal. This subject has been ably treated by several authors, and I shall, in my future work, discuss some of the checks at considerable length, more especially in regard to the feral animals of South America. Here I will make only a few remarks, just to recall to the reader's mind some of the chief points. Eggs or very young animals seem generally to suffer most, but this is not invariably the case. With plants there is a vast destruction of seeds, but, from some observations which I have made, I believe that it is the seedlings which suffer most from germinating in ground already thickly stocked with other plants. Seedlings, also, are destroyed in vast numbers by various enemies; for instance, on a piece of ground three feet long and two wide, dug and cleared, and where there could be no choking from other plants, I marked all the seedling of our native weeds as they came up, and out of the 357 no less than 295 were destroyed, chiefly by slugs and insects. If turf which has long been mown, and the case would be the same with turf closely browsed by quadrupeds, be let to grow, the more vigorous plants gradually kill the less vigorous, though fully grown, plants; thus out of twenty species growing on a little plot of turf (three feet by four) nine species perished from the other species being allowed to grow up freely. (Darwin C: *op. cit.,* Chapter III. The Struggle for Existence.)

The second means of condensation, excising superfluous words, can strikingly reduce the bulk of a draft. Sometimes half of the words in a phrase can be dropped out without any loss of meaning.

evacuate [the contents of] the cyst

The following [is a list of] drugs [which] depress . . .

A phrase may be reducible to a single word.

 results in a weakening of → weakens
 There are some occasions when → Occasionally

Deleting words and phrases calls for at least as much care and judgment as substituting short ones for long. Do not mistake needed connectives and transitional material for cobwebs, or sacrifice accuracy by such crude ellipses as *aortic murmur* for *aortic valvular murmur, beta blockade* for *beta-adrenergic blockade* and *pregnant serum* for *the serum of pregnant women.* These may pass in speech but they are too clipped for formal writing. It is a delusion that clarity and readability are improved by dense constructions like *distal renal tubule proton secretion impairment;* beware of precipitating such semantic log-jams.

The cryptic terseness found in much technical writing less often results from carelessness or laziness than from deliberate but misguided efforts at compression. Extreme condensation of material is unnatural and injurious to the texture and rhythm of English prose. Moreover, it forces the reader into a state of exaggerated attention which rapidly becomes fatiguing. Since the absorption and assimilation of written matter demands a certain minimum of connection and reinforcement, and a little breathing-space between enunciations of major points, undue terseness diminishes both the reader's comprehension and his comfort. A telegram is a model of conciseness, but no one wants to read telegrams all day.

The technical writer must not take seriously everything that is preached in the name of conciseness. Some authorities, overreacting to the kind of muddy verbiage that clouds meaning and mesmerizes the reader into inattention, have flown to the opposite extreme and advocated baldness or baby-talk.

The Elements of Style, by William Strunk, Jr., a book of less than a hundred pages, should be read and reread by anyone who aspires to write for publication. (First issued in 1918; currently in print in a revised version edited by E. B. White. New York, The Macmillan Company, 1959; paperback, 1962.) *The Elements of Style,* originally prepared as a classbook for an English course at Cornell University, has achieved worldwide fame as a practical guide to a clean and vigorous writing style. If Strunk had a fault it was his relentless insistence on brevity and succinctness, an understandable crotchet in a man who spent much of his time reading the literary productions of college students. In his zeal for getting rid of weeds, Strunk sometimes seems to uproot and kill the flowers as well.

The mania for brevity often drives a writer into frank inaccuracy by tempting him to understatement, overstatement or unwarranted generalization. G. K. Chesterton was rather severe on American journalists of the 1930s because of the ways in which they pared and twisted the English language, particularly in headlines.

> This is one of the evils produced by that passion for compression and compact information which possesses so many ingenious minds in America. Everybody can see how an entirely new system of grammar, syntax, and even language has been invented to fit the brevity of headlines. Such brevity, so far from being the soul of wit, is even the death of meaning; and certainly the death of logic. (Chesterton GK: *GK's Weekly* [London], May 2, 1931.)

In the 1940s Rudolf Flesch propounded the doctrine that readability can be reduced to a mathematical formula based on words per sentence and syllables per hundred words. (See Flesch R: *The Art of Readable Writing*. New York, Harper & Row, 1949; reissued 1974. For a review of this work see King LS: Toward better writing. *JAMA* 229:852, 1974.) Since Flesch's book came on the scene just after World War II, when America was in the raptures of a second technological revolution, the public avidly swallowed his mechanistic theory of communication. Though his advocacy of this twentieth-century gift of tongues was less than brilliant (for he was rash enough to practice what he preached), his promise of instant and universal intelligibility found a ready clientele among free-lance journalists, advertising copywriters and kindred hacks. (Flesch was not the only rhetorician to develop a readability formula, or even the first. For a detailed study see Klare GR: *The Measurement of Readability*. Ames, Iowa, Iowa State University Press, 1963.)

"In striving too earnestly after conciseness," confessed Horace, "I run headlong into inarticulateness." Short words and short sentences do not necessarily ensure either readability or clarity. Indeed, they do not even lead to economy of language except when platitudes and trifles are being uttered. Since a condensed and monosyllabic style cannot efficiently express abstract concepts or closely reasoned analyses and deductions, the writer is forced into wasteful and tedious repetition, which vastly increases the number of words needed to do the job. Instead of a clean, concentrated style this kind of "brevity" generates a leisurely and disorganized verbosity.

The widely differing standards of conciseness set up by Strunk and Flesch may both serve very well to trim the padding and froth from amateur fiction and to curtail the syntactic exuberance of the neophyte essayist, journalist or advertising writer, but they cannot be applied very strictly to scientific exposition. Though conciseness is undoubtedly a virtue in technical writing, it must never become an end in itself. The basic issue is not bulk but concentration, not length but design. The ideal of verbal economy lies somewhere between boring the reader to death and assailing him with an unremitting staccato of ideas.

GRAPHIC MATERIALS

Some structures, techniques and relationships are so intricate or abstruse that the attempt to describe them with words alone is folly. A surgery text without illustrations or a textbook of physiology without graphs and tables would not be of much use. Early in the course of preparing material for publication you should determine whether tables, graphs, drawings or photographs (including photomicrographs and x-rays) will add to the clarity of your presentation.

Selecting and arranging graphic materials deserves as much attention as writing the text. Unless your drawings, graphs and photographs are of high professional quality no reputable journal will print them. They must be kept simple, clear and free of irrelevant or distracting detail. Tables should add something, not merely duplicate or recapitulate the text. The caption (or legend) of an illustration should be concise but informative, and in the case of a photomicrograph it should tell the magnification and staining method.

Be sure that your name and the title of the paper appear on the back of each illustration submitted. The designation of each ("Figure 1," "Table D") and its caption should also be written on the back or firmly attached. The top of each illustration should be clearly marked with an arrow on the back. Never write or type directly on the reverse side of a photographic print or ECG tracing. Instead, place the required information on a label and attach it to the back. Do not use an adhesive with a volatile solvent, which may discolor photographic inks or warp paper.

Each clinical photograph should be accompanied by the patient's written consent to publication, even if it is impossible to recognize him in the picture. Follow the publisher's directions for photographs of minors; usually the consent of both parents is required.

Davidson's *Guide to Medical Writing* (New York, The Ronald Press Co, 1957), regrettably out of print, contains valuable information on the preparation of graphic materials. Though medical illustration and medical photography are not promising fields for amateur endeavor, an excellent recent work, *Technical Illustrating* by G. E. Morris (Englewood Cliffs, NJ, Prentice-Hall, Inc, 1975) can be highly recommended. Several fine monographs on medical photography are published by Charles C. Thomas, Springfield, Illinois, and by the Eastman Kodak Company, Rochester, New York.

Reproduction techniques may badly blur the contrasts and alter the colors of clinical photographs and photomicrographs. It is not unusual for the printed version of a radiograph to appear perfectly normal, though the full-sized original contains conspicuous abnormalities. Printing a clinical photograph frequently "cures" skin lesions plainly visible in the original. Review previous issues of the *Journal* to which you propose to submit your paper so as to judge the printer's ability to reproduce your graphic materials. Insist upon seeing either page proofs or a photocopy of the printer's layout to verify that illustrations have been inserted right-side-up, that transparencies have not been reversed, and that captions have been placed where they belong. Misleading graphic materials are worse than none at all.

CLARITY: PRACTICAL GUIDELINES

1. Be literal, concrete and explicit, selecting the most exact and precise word to express each idea.
2. Revise your work carefully and repeatedly so that every sentence is perfectly clear on the first reading.
3. Emphasize major points by repetition, exemplification, analogy or any other technique that makes them striking and memorable.
4. In revising, remove unnecessary words and phrases, and replace long words with short ones when possible.
5. Select graphic materials with care, keep them simple and relevant, and be sure that they add to the worth of the finished piece instead of detracting from it.

REFERENCES

Buchanan RE, Gibbons NE: *Bergey's Manual of Determinative Bacteriology,* ed 8. Baltimore, Williams & Wilkins Co, 1974.
Cowan ST: *A Dictionary of Microbial Taxonomic Usage.* Edinburgh, Oliver & Boyd, 1968.
Current Medical Information and Terminology, ed 4. Chicago, American Medical Association, 1971.
Current Procedural Terminology, ed 4. Chicago, American Medical Association, 1977.

Page C: *The International System of Units* (SI). Washington, US Government Printing Office, 1974.

Standard Metric Practice Guide (ASTM E380-72). Philadelphia, American Society for Testing and Materials, 1972.

USAN and the USP Dictionary of Drug Names. Rockville, Md, The United States Pharmacopoeial Convention, Inc, 1976.

Vawter SM, DeForest RE: The international metric system and medicine. *JAMA* 218:723-726, 1971.

9

Readability

By the readability of writing we mean its capacity not merely to be read, but to be read with ease, comfort and even pleasure. There are practical as well as esthetic reasons for trying to keep technical writing light, interesting and attractive. A smooth and pleasant style enhances the reader's understanding and retention of the material. Moreover, besides those who read out of necessity or duty, another group, perhaps larger than the first, may be drawn to read an appealingly written paper.

Intelligibility and readability complement and reinforce each other. In striving for a fluid style that moves smoothly along, the writer must perforce avoid bringing his reader up with a jerk in the middle of a sentence to untie a syntactic knot or distill a meaning diluted by excess verbiage. In other words, readable writing is of necessity clear and intelligible writing. There is a certain natural beauty in anything that functions with precision and economy, be it a blacksmith or a racehorse, a punch-press or a paragraph.

The key to readable writing is sustaining the reader's interest, good will and receptivity. This seems so self-evident that we may well wonder why medical literature is so often stilted, dry, monotonous, abstract and impersonal. One answer that promptly suggests itself is that medical writing is intended to impart information, not to entertain. The author is so taken up with accuracy, clarity and objectivity that he almost instinctively shies away from modes of expression that are meant to impress, amuse or charm. And yet, as I hope to show, there is a broad middle ground between the dull and distant tone of a directory or compendium and the meretricious glitter of the popular press.

A second reason for the dreariness of much medical writing is the absence of any strong motive for trying to make it otherwise. Medical writing is seldom a lucrative undertaking, and even the top-selling texts do not make their authors wealthy. Writing that is mandated by the law of "publish or perish" is often mere drudgery from which the author can expect neither glory nor profit. And of course a publisher of medical textbooks or a journal editor takes more interest in an author's credentials and the accuracy and clarity of his presentation than in its grace or eloquence.

Thirdly, the subject matter of much medical writing possesses enough intellectual appeal to attract readers and to ensure that many of them will plod on to the bitter end even at the cost of some discomfort. That is why a medical writer with special experience or authority can command an attentive audience even though he refuses to do his readers the elementary courtesy of learning to write. His fondness for jargon and high-flown phraseology, and his crass ineptitude at putting sentences together, may rob his writings of charm as well as clarity, but they will be read all the same if the germ of meaning buried in them is worth digging out, or if the author's reputation even suggests that it might be.

Admittedly, a medical writer cannot show much originality in his choice or handling of technical terms: they are already chosen for him, and their meanings are fixed. If he wishes to avoid tedious repetition he may have to decide between an inexact synonym and a cumbersome circumlocution. But the bulk of the words he uses are plain English, and besides being conventional and arbitrary symbols for units of meaning, these are also the hues and shades, the cadences and harmonies of an art form. By selecting his words judiciously and arranging them skillfully, the proficient writer works a magical effect with words which far transcends their bare meaning.

Though "bare meaning" may seem the only proper motive for scientific exposition, even the technical writer must foresee and reckon with the reader's reaction to the manner and style of his presentation, as well as to its burden of facts. It is not enough for the writer to know perfectly the definitions of the words he uses; he must also cultivate a feeling for their color, weight and texture.

CADENCE

By cadence we mean the tempo and rhythm of writing. If these terms suggest a piece of music or a dramatic recitation, that is exactly what they should do. The careful writer puts words together with his ears as well as his eyes on the result. Remember that letters are phonetic symbols, and that writing is a representation of speech. The reader hears in his mind the sound of what he reads. No writer ever pleased a large audience without coming to terms with that fact.

An example will make this clearer. If in reading you come to the word *tears*, and suppose that it means the secretion of the lacrimal gland, your mind registers the pronunciation *teerz*. On discovering in the next sentence that the reference is actually to lacerations, you experience a momentary cerebral arrest: you find it necessary to backtrack and erase, so to speak, the wrong pronunciation before proceeding.

Achieving a pleasing cadence really has very little to do with the avoidance of such phonetic miscues. On the positive and esthetic side, let us hear Robert Louis Stevenson—no dull theorist or obscure rhetorician but the author of popular novels which can be read with pleasure a century after they were written.

> . . . Between the implication and the evolution of the sentence there should be a satisfying equipoise of sound; for nothing more often disappoints the ear than a sentence solemnly and sonorously prepared, and hastily and weakly finished. Nor should the balance be too striking and exact, for the one rule is to be infinitely various; to interest, to disappoint, to surprise, and yet still to gratify; to be ever changing, as it were, the stitch, and yet still to give the effect of an ingenious neatness. (Stevenson RL: On style in literature, its technical elements. *The Contemporary Review* [London], April, 1885.)

Are we to take seriously the assertion that the sole means of producing a pleasing sound in prose is to produce a constantly various one? We do not find a siren more melodious than a hymn-tune, though it may arouse livelier emotions. To understand Stevenson's rule of infinite variety we must recall the five species of phonetic pattern in literature, as classified by the art of poetics.

ALLITERATION (the repetition of an initial consonant): positive pressure, cut and clamp, serial serum samples

CONSONANCE (the recurrence of a consonant or consonant cluster): apparently parous, vasa vasorum, tibial tubercle

ASSONANCE (the recurrence of a vowel sound): gross sodium overload, three feeble squeaks

RHYME (the recurrence of end sounds): dry eye, heart cart, numb thumb, deliver to the liver

RHYTHM (the fall of accents): *This* is a *case* of ru*bel*la in *which* the arth*ri*tis ap*peared* in the *pro*drome and *led* us at *first* to sus*pect* a rheu*matic* or *rheuma*toid *pro*cess.

A prose style that seeks to achieve its effects by a deliberate cultivation of these patterns seems mannered and grotesque. Though such tricks may be effective in some genres other than poetry, technical exposition is not one of them. A medical text written in the style of John Lyly or Thomas Carlyle would probably be a phenomenal flop.

Because alliteration, consonance, assonance and rhyme all consist in conspicuous repetition of sounds, the art of writing comfortable and unobtrusive prose demands that they be carefully avoided. Because a regularly repetitive pattern of accents, as in the example above, is ludicrous and distracting, the fastidious writer breaks up the rhythm of his words and phrases into as random a pattern as possible.

Now we see that Stevenson, discriminating critic and inspired choreographer of words that he was, knew perfectly well what he was talking about when he identified variety as the "one rule." How is variety to be achieved? Let us consult him again.

> Each phrase of each sentence, like an air or a recitative in music, should be so artfully compounded out of long and short, out of accented and unaccented, as to gratify the sensual ear. And of this the ear is the sole judge. It is impossible to lay down laws. Even in our accentual and rhythmic language no analysis can find the beauty of a verse; how much less, then, of those phrases, such as prose is built of, which obey no law but to be lawless and yet to please? (*ibid.*)

The writer must cultivate an ear for a pleasing variety of sound, and write to please that ear. The words and phrases of a well-turned sentence, like each successive note of an Irving Berlin melody, engender a mild and pleasurable surprise, coupled with the immediate realization that any other word or any other sequence would probably have yielded a less suitable cadence. Not that the talent of a genius is needed to produce a pleasing paragraph. Words are more variegated and more tractable than musical tones, and their proper disposition with respect to sound as well as meaning comes naturally to the practiced writer.

The beginning writer must learn to avoid both phonetic blemishes and the tiresome and aimless repetition of words and sounds. Jingles or unwanted rhymes creep inevitably into everyone's writing, and must be carefully weeded out during revision. Rhyming end sounds ("usually only slightly unsightly") get past editors with distressing frequency. Beginning sounds that jingle ("initial inciting incident") are only slightly less annoying.

> *The objective of taping an injured ankle is the prevention of inadvertent eversion and inversion of the joint.

Here in the space of seven words we have the prefix *in-* three times and the syllable *ver* three times.

The means of breaking up these awkward phonetic clusters are obvious: substitute another word for one or more of the jingling ones, or move them further apart. The writer's ingenuity may be sorely taxed when he must compose an extended passage in which certain technical terms inevitably recur together—for instance, a comparison of leiomyoma and leiomyosarcoma. A pronoun or a synonym can be substituted for one of the terms as long as the meaning is perfectly clear.

> These occur at an earlier age than leiomyosarcoma and do not metastasize.
> Evidence of invasion of normal tissue differentiates leiomyosarcoma from benign tumor.

Once the pattern of comparison is established, it may suffice to use only one of the terms.

> Leiomyosarcoma is much more prone to severe hemorrhage.

The repetition of a sound must be distinguished from the repetition of a word. As I discussed in an earlier chapter, word echo can be used deliberately to focus or maintain the reader's attention or reinforce his awareness of a context or viewpoint. By contrast, aimless echoing of words bores and distracts.

> *follow the following plan
> *produced by production of
> *determine response to a determined amount of exercise
> *a means of improving patient compliance in these patients

Particularly maladroit is the careless repetition of a word in different connotations.

> *Statistical data are of little value to the physician who must evaluate measured blood pressure values in the individual.

The unwanted echo *value . . . values* is rendered still more disagreeable by the intrusion of *evaluate.*

> *The recognition of the kidney and the pancreas as endocrine as well as as exocrine glands came later.

Here we have *as* four times in eighteen words. This is not ungrammatical; it is too grammatical, for all but the strictest purists would condone ommission of the last *as*. The reader of such a sentence is struck not by its grammar but by its eccentricty and repulsiveness, and that is what the writer must correct.

Whatever means you choose for avoiding an unwanted repetition, be sure that the result is really an improvement. A common failing among inexperienced writers is to reach for variety by concocting a hash of bizarre inversions and inappropriate surrogate words which distract, confuse and annoy. Students in many high-school and college composition courses are still taught that repetition of commonplace words must be avoided at all costs. For *is* they are encouraged to substitute verbs with more clout, though the choice often falls on some equally static abstraction like *exists, constitutes* or *represents*. This style of teaching has given rise to the delusion that a crazy quilt of synonyms is vigorous, racy writing. Second-rate journalists have done much to perpetuate this specious standard of eloquence, and second-rate editors commonly impose it on material submitted to them for revision.

Perhaps no book besides the Bible has been so often misapplied and put to wrong uses as Roget's *Thesaurus*. This work, compiled by a nineteenth-century English physician, groups synonyms and related words in exactly one thousand categories. It is intended as a synopsis for quick reference, where the writer can see at a glance most of the choices available to express his idea. Though valuable in its way, the *Thesaurus* contains no definitions. Its user must therefore know exactly what the listed words mean, or learn this from the proper source, before he chooses one and puts it on paper.

A high-school pupil may be forgiven for believing that he can add color and pungency to his writing by pulling words indiscriminately out of Roget and stringing together such a hodge-podge of garbage as the following.

> *Festinating up to the myrmidon, I catechized him as to the situation of the arena wherein the emulation was to be adjudicated, hurtled there with celerity, and disembarked precisely *a tempo.*

However, an adult writing for publication who produces material in this vein deserves a flogging.

So extreme an example as this of obsession with synonyms is not likely to pass across a medical editor's desk. There is nevertheless a tendency among technical writers to avoid repeating a word by substituting a synonym whose strangeness or inexactness renders it more conspicuous than repetition of the original would be. Thus, the author of a two-part presentation on ocular infection shies away from the obvious headings and gives us jargon instead: *Extraocular Involvement* and *Intraocular Entities.*

Notice how clumsy and disjointed the first sentence below seems, because the writer would not choose one word for a test result and stick to it.

> *Of 120 patients with proved pulmonary embolism, 18% had elevation of serum lactate dehydrogenase *value,* elevation of serum bilirubin *concentration,* and a normal serum glutamic oxalacetic transaminase *level.*
>
> *Recent epidemiologic studies indicate that populations on a high sodium intake have a higher blood pressure than patients on a low sodium intake.

The needless shift from *populations* to *patients* in the second sentence is worse than distracting: it introduces an element of confusion by falsely suggesting that a distinction is being drawn between persons using salt at will ("populations") and those under treatment with a low-sodium diet ("patients").

In these examples the restless compulsion to constantly vary a term has created, at worst, a misleading and annoying lack of parallelism, but sometimes it results in inaccuracy. The writer of a paper on inflammatory disease of the large bowel wants to warn his readers against mistaking amebic colitis for ulcerative colitis. Dreading the repetition of *colitis,* he writes, "Amebic colitis must not be mistaken for ulcerative disease," which is nonsense, since amebic colitis is itself an ulcerative disease.

BALANCE AND PHRASING

Besides the phonetic cadence of writing there is a semantic cadence, a systole and diastole of meaning corresponding to the ebb and flow of the reader's attention, and closely akin to what an actor or comedian calls timing. The composition of a sentence, like that of a picture, ought to have a balance, a satisfying disposition of parts around a center of gravity. As in painting, photography and sculpture, this balance depends on a host of ill-defined and largely subjective features, which, however hard they may be to isolate and describe, are nevertheless plainly discernible to all but the most obtuse. The neglect of this balance generally arises not from obtuseness but from an indifference to the reader's comfort and pleasure, and a resultant failure to consider the esthetics of writing.

In every sentence of whatever structure, the opening words create a frame of reference, a psychological setting in which the reader will perceive and interpret everything that follows. Because any pronounced shift in this setting is awkward, confusing and distracting to the reader, it can seldom if ever be justified on rhetorical grounds. That is why grammar and composition books so consistently and vehemently condemn the practice of opening a sentence with a dangling participle.

> *Using Burger's technique, four rats survived adrenalectomy for more than six months.

The ideal sentence comes quickly to the point. Though a brief introductory passage sometimes improves clarity or lends a pleasing variety, a sentence with a lengthy preamble seems top-heavy and long-winded. The serious and attentive reader does not need a running start to get into the core and substance of each sentence. If he did, the common practice of launching a statement in the realm of the abstract would not help much. "The most frequently observed difference between A and B is in particle size" not only starts off in the abstract, it stays there. Why not just say "A particles are usually bigger than B particles"?

Too often a writer employs a vague or hackneyed introductory formula to draw the unsuspecting reader into the midst of an absurdity or a non sequitur. Starting a sentence with "As everyone knows" or "It is generally agreed" and finishing it with a highly dubious or controversial assertion is like putting blinders on a horse and backing it over a cliff.

The end of a sentence is no less crucial than the beginning. Even in sentences that are not laid out in periodic form—the great majority—the end position must be respected and handled with care. A sentence is not like a windup toy that proceeds steadily from a state of full energy at the start to one of inertia at the end. Each half of the sentence ought to bear an approximately equal burden of meaning, so that they balance neatly around an imaginary node or caesura near the middle. When properly poised, a sentence has a tail-light, a last intellectual fillip to the reader. Ending with a weak prepositional phrase, as in the following example, gives the reader a jolt of disappointment.

> *Protective circulatory adjustments occur rapidly in acute blood loss, but they have a limited power of compensation, and they can usually correct losses of about 30% of the total blood volume at most.

In rhetoric, the term *climax* preserves its classical meaning (Greek, *ladder*) and refers to the whole of an ascending series, not just its highest point or culmination. A sense of climax is critical to the proper disposition of a series. Generally speaking, a series whose members vary in magnitude or importance should ascend steadily. If you write that the patient had "four fractured ribs, a ruptured spleen, a pneumothorax and an abrasion of the knee," you inflict an anticlimax on the reader. The abrupt drop in level lets him fall flat, and whether he reacts with amusement or annoyance the general result is a loss of effectiveness. Similarly, it is so natural to list drowsiness, confusion, delirium, stupor, coma and death in that order that any other would seem eccentric.

Sentences constructed without due attention to balance and climax cannot fail to induce malaise and indigestion. Much the same observation may be made about the design of paragraphs. Even when every sentence after the first one is a simple statement of fact, exemplifying or demonstrating what is set down in the first, the concluding words of a paragraph ought to round off the whole neatly instead of leaving the reader hanging. But beware of adorning the end of a paragraph with empty verbiage just to give it the right look on the page, or the right balance to the ear. The ideal is an intellectual as well as an auditory rounding off, not a final sentence composed entirely of inert ingredients.

> *. . . The incidence of murmurs in children between the ages of 11 and 19 ranges from 32 to 44%. Organic lesions account for a very small fraction of these murmurs. Most murmurs are the result of hemodynamic factors which produce sounds of sufficient intensity to be audible to the human ear.

Padding is tiresome enough in a novel, but in technical writing it is simply intolerable.

Another feature that is vital to a comfortable writing style is skillful phrasing. I refer here to a phrase not in its grammatical meaning but in the broader sense of any group of words, whether two or 32, which are meant to be taken together. Phrasing in music depends on the length of the violinist's bow (ultimately on the length of his arm) and on the vital capacity of the oboist's or the tenor's lungs. The amount of information which the mind can grasp at one time is also subject to physiologic limits. A sentence is a mental mouthful: if it is too short it will disappoint the reader, if too long it will choke him.

The beginning writer tends to write in short and simple sentences, just as he might dictate.

    *Digitalis can produce every known kind of cardiac arrhythmia. It can do this by altering either formation or conduction of impulses. It may alter both at the same time. Cardiac arrhythmias of one kind or another can be expected to occur in about 90% of patients with digitalis toxicity. Such a patient may have a combination of arrhythmias. He may also change from one arrhythmia to another within a single ECG tracing.

Once he begins to get the knack of composition, he may veer to the other extreme.

    *Digitalis-induced arrhythmias, arising from disturbances of either formation or conduction of impulses, or both, may be of any known type and may occur in as high as 90% of patients with digitalis toxicity, some of whom may display a combination of arrhythmias or may even change from one arrhythmia to another within a single ECG tracing.

Sentence-sense, a feel for the amount of matter that will fit comfortably into a sentence, is developed only by practice, specifically by careful revision of one's own work some time after it has been written. Faulty sentence-sense is a bugbear with editors, and dooms many an otherwise worthy manuscript to rejection.

I have spoken already of variation in sound patterns. Syntactic patterns need to vary a little, too. It is not always feasible to arrange sentences so that long and short ones alternate in pleasingly random fashion. An unbroken string of long sentences is less apt to produce restlessness and ennui than a series of short ones. This is fortunate, since technical writing of necessity contains a high proportion of compound and complex sentences. An occasional very short sentence not only breaks up the monotony but, as I have shown elsewhere, can neatly focus attention by crystallizing an idea or concept.

In the last analysis, sentence length exerts less influence on the reader's comfort than sentence structure. A long succession of sentences built on an unvarying subject-verb-complement framework creates a soporific monotony. Moreover, such a series will often be found to lack adequate correlation and emphasis. The grammatical inversions described in Chapter 7 as ways to show transition and achieve emphasis can also serve to vary sentence structure. As noted there, such devices as the passive voice and introductory expletives must be used with discretion and restraint.

VIGOR

Why does one piece of writing live and breathe and strike fire from the flint of the reader's intellect, while another drags itself ponderously and wearily along under a leaden pall of dullness? Though I cannot isolate and analyze the quintessential principle that sets apart the writer of talent and genius from his uninspired and unread contemporaries, I can list some of the ways in which his work differs from theirs.

A writer of intellectual power puts something of that power into his work: it is vivid, energetic, forceful. A positive tone enlivens writing because it is direct, tangible, and seems to give something to the reader. By contrast, a negative tone is indirect, abstract, and seems to take something away. The compelling writer chooses the positive over the negative, the concrete over the abstract, the specific over the general and the active over the passive.

Vigorous writing is challenging, thought-provoking and original, not anonymous, perfunctory and predictable. It glows not with the ersatz vivacity of the *Reader's Digest* but with a genuine spark of the writer's own intellectual fire. A strong and independent spirit is never content to parrot cliches, whether of word, phrase or idea, no matter how apt and accurate they may seem. Robust writing is distinctive: it bears the stamp of the author's personality, and eschews sterile, dull and soporific formulas.

The writer of power shuns feeble and lifeless terms like *involve* and *situation;* he deals in real things and events and he calls them by their first names, not by types and figures. He certainly is never caught writing eyewash like *multilevel therapeutic model* or *prototypal entity.*

Lively, articulate writing puts across its main ideas with nouns and verbs. A writer who depends on adjectives, adverbs and subordinate clauses to convey the bulk of his meaning raises an edifice of gingerbread on a foundation of quicksand. Until sometime in the last century, an unconscious nominalism ruled English prose composition: strong and vivid nouns worked shoulder to shoulder with prosaic and colorless verbs *(is, has, does)*. Whereas modern British usage preserves much of this character, American English, influenced no doubt by writers like Mark Twain and O. Henry, displays an ardent and sometimes unfortunate fondness for the colorful or metaphorical verb. The best technical exposition steers a middle course, which comes easier to the writer who has cultivated a familiarity with clean, comfortable prose.

Nothing injects vigor and dash into writing like a judicious sprinkling of short, vivid, exact words. Anglo-Saxon derivatives are usually best suited for this purpose: *unfold* means the same as *develop, turn around*

the same as *revolve, give* the same as *impart,* but in each case the
Latinate word seems effete and effeminate beside its Anglo-Saxon
synonym. Note, too, that the Romance word is usually longer. *Alteration*
seems more ponderous and pretentious than *change, conceal* than *mask,*
demonstrate than *show.* The longer words are all of respectable pedigree
and steady habits, and each of them has its place, but the shorter ones
are very often preferable.

A further difference worth noting between Anglo-Saxon words and
those of Greek and Latin origin is that the latter are apt to be more
bookish and abstract. The dissimilarities in vocabulary between speech
and writing, alluded to in an earlier chapter, are perhaps greater in
English than in any other modern language, and one of the main
grounds of distinction is that the language of the pen is much richer in
words of Mediterranean birth than the language of the tongue. We have
no choice but to use terms of classical origin when we want to talk
about, for example, inflammation of the esophagus: *fire in the weasand*
just would not do at all. But in everyday speech even the pedants among
us use a high proportion of Anglo-Saxon words, keeping their formi-
dable stock of Greek and Latin derivatives shut away with the ink. Since
words seldom spoken are likely to seem stale and moldy when met with
in print, forceful writing holds them to a minimum.

A well-chosen metaphor can energize technical prose and wake up the
reader.

> The suprascapular and transverse cervical arteries clamp the
>   phrenic nerve to the scalenus anticus muscle.
> It may sometimes be possible to snake a smaller catheter inside the
>   larger past the obstruction.

Notice how *clamp* and *snake* lend color and vividness to these sentences,
shedding a glow of life over their neighbors like diamonds set among
humbler stones. We cannot, after all, replace technical terms with anything more brisk or pungent without straying into inaccuracy and
obscurity. But the judicious insertion of a single colorful metaphor
among these mundane, workaday words gives sparkle and freshness to
the whole passage.

The best and most engaging writing has a sort of warmth or geniality,
a quality which assures the reader that there is another human being
across the void of time and space. Good writing is not a monolog but a
conversation between writer and reader. Never lose your awareness of
your audience, its capacities, its temperament, its expectations. A novelist
or a musician who did so would soon have no audience. You must
commune with your reader, not just jabber at him. Do not commit the

blunder of playing to the grandstand, couching your ideas in the arcane mumbo-jumbo of a superspecialty to impress a handful of readers while alienating all the rest.

Warmth in writing comes across in many subtle ways: in the respect which the writer shows for the reader, in his evident enthusiasm for his subject, in the little glimpses he gives of his own personality, individuality and good nature.

> The reflex hammer should be gripped firmly and swung smartly and decisively through a substantial arc, say 60°, of which the examiner's wrist joint forms the center of rotation. A satisfactory hammer needs a certain weight, of which the usual medical supply house article falls short. The "hammer" that I have used for the past eleven years is an eight-inch length of solid brass curtain-rod covered with rubber tubing.

The last sentence brings us closer to the writer, tells us more about him, sells him and his ideas to us more persuasively than all the rest of his paper together. The personal touch must not, of course, be overdone, or permitted to degenerate into a patronizing or insolently familiar manner.

"Why," asked Horace, "should we not spice up the lesson with a dash of humor?" In two thousand years no one has even tried to find an answer. When we consider the importance to the physician of a cheerful and genial temperament, which can ease patients' sufferings, lighten the burden of work and smooth relationships with colleagues, it seems surprising and regrettable that a little gentle humor does not more often find its way into medical literature.

Admittedly, medical writing does not offer a wide scope for humor. Ribaldry and sarcasm are always out of place. A paper on multiple sclerosis or teenage suicide would be marred, not enhanced, by any attempt at wit. But a hint of quiet drollery may sometimes enliven material which instead of being lugubrious is merely dull. Nothing makes technical exposition so boring and unpalatable as an undue gravity of tone.

"Don't pull on the umbilical cord," said one of my teachers, and immediately hammered home his point with an Irish bull: "You may pull it off, and then you won't have anything to pull out the placenta with." As every good teacher knows, humor can be of immense value in emphasizing an idea. A writer who wanted to underscore the importance of the rectal examination made good use of a pun when he concluded his paper with the advice that the physician "*digitalize* every patient." A vivid simile may also reinforce a message while keeping the tone light and interesting.

It is said that pityriasis rosea will fade completely after systemic administration of adrenal steroid, but this seems rather like going after ants with dynamite.

Humor and figurative language must be administered in small doses. A flippant or bantering tone undermines the whole effect of technical writing. The intelligent reader recoils in disgust from fustian drivel like the following:

> *Abandoning these superficial haunts, the vessel plunges boldly into the depths of the last-named fossa, courses inferiorly in familiar association with its faithful venae comites, and at length emerges triumphant . . .

and from mere silliness like this:

> *During the first 48 hours the patient may experience chills, fever and a slight cough, with a pinch of nausea thrown in for good measure.

If there is anyone capable of writing a whole paper or book along these lines, would you be surprised to learn that he pours champagne and ketchup over his corn flakes every morning?

No matter how picturesque his language or how piquant his wit, the technical writer must never forget what he is doing and allow his presentation to degenerate into pure entertainment. Neither should he surround his subject with a spurious aura of tension and melodrama. The popular novelist may find it expedient to manufacture atmosphere in this earnest, hamming way, but the manner and tone of technical writing must always be suited to and subservient to the matter.

It is possible to write vigorous, appealing, even amusing prose and still preserve a due formality and decorum. It is not possible to write slang like *heading up the lab team* or *now for the bad news* without descending to sloppy informality. A correctly formed taste complements vividness and humor while keeping them in check; it ensures that the writer will not sew purple patches on burlap and call if finery, or try to juice up his paragraphs with forced and mirthless jocularity.

Not only does good taste protect the writer from conspicuous eccentricity, but it also adds a final polish to his style. Tasteful prose is nearly always pleasant to read. Indeed, the very foundation of good taste in writing is an intimate familiarity with good literature. One who does not himself derive pleasure from reading can hardly be expected to give pleasure to others through his writing.

THE TITLE AND OPENING PASSAGE

Since the title is the handle by which your paper will be retrieved from the vast storehouse of the medical literature, it ought to be truthful, specific and distinctive. If it has all three of these qualities it should prove well able to perform its basic job of identifying and introducing the paper as it first appears in print.

Though the title can hardly be counted on to tell the whole truth, it must tell nothing but the truth. As it stands in the *Cumulated Index Medicus* or in any other bibliography it should give an accurate idea of what is in the paper. There is just enough ambiguity in *following, associated with* and *secondary to* that these prepositions should be rigorously excluded from titles. If a relation is purely temporal, *after* is the preposition of choice (unless, indeed, the relation is more naturally expressed by *before*). If the paper establishes a casual connection, *due to* or *caused by* is the appropriate term.

Even if *The Dermatologist's Dilemma* represents the topic of a paper truthfully, it conveys too little information. Though such a title may attract many readers at the time of publication, it damns the paper to eventual oblivion. *A New Treatment for Snakebite* holds something back, making an unnecessary mystery of what the treatment is. *Radioactive Quartz in Snakebite* is better, since it gives a fuller idea of the subject treated and incidentally suggests a second heading under which the paper can be indexed. But if the new treatment is effective only in cobra bite, this title is still not specific enough.

Making a title distinctive may pose special problems. The number of feasible variations on *The Treatment of Hypertension with Propranolol* is limited. A subtitle may be of use in distinguishing your research report from forty others on the same subject: *Propranolol in Hypertension. Long-term Study in Inmates of a Women's Prison.* The social status of the subjects is not germane to the study and therefore does not belong in the main title, but it is perfectly proper to bring it into the subtitle.

Generally the more concise the title, the better. However, the writer should follow the usual practice of the journal to which he submits his paper. Very long, comprehensive and explicit titles are currently in vogue in some of the specialty journals. Though cumbersome, these certainly provide adequate compass for attaining the three ideals of veracity, specificity and distinctiveness. In no case, however, should your title contain a single word that is not absolutely necessary. In *An Investigation to Measure the Efficacy of Fructose in Orf* all but the last three words are inert and superfluous.

Do not underestimate the importance of your opening passage. Customarily the introductory paragraph, like the overture of an opera, is written after the rest of the work is done. This is not objectionable as long as the job receives due care and attention. Though the first sentence may impart less information than any other in the whole paper, in one sense it is the most critical, since it is the first one that the reader will see. A dreary and discordant overture bodes no good for the opera-goer who sits out the performance. A clumsy opening sentence may impress the reader as a preview of coming distractions and send him off in search of better things elsewhere.

Your opening ought to seize and hold the reader's attention, give him an accurate foretaste of both your material and your style of presenting it, and move into the subject quickly. The reader is only human. If your opening fails to attract him to read further, you may as well not write further. But beware of trying to tantalize him by propounding a riddle or asking a question at the outset. Leave such cheap trickery to the slick magazines.

Above all, avoid a lengthy preamble, an apologetic or self-laudatory tone, and a posture of false humility. Humorous anecdotes or reminiscences may serve very well to start a lecture or an address but they are bad taste in formal writing. An opening like "More years ago than I care to remember . . ." puts the seal of death on a paper.

Probably the most effective method of writing an introductory passage is to sum up in a sentence or two the subject of the paper and then carefully refine this material until it is as concise and appealing as you can make it. There is no objection to a bold metaphor here, or a trace of humor, as long as accuracy and good taste are not violated.

READABILITY: PRACTICAL GUIDELINES

1. Make a conscious effort to keep your presentation interesting and attractive.
2. Avoid expressions that are unduly negative, distant, dry or abstract.
3. Balance your sentences carefully and pay attention to phrasing and climax.
4. Choose words and phrases that are fresh, vivid and forceful.
5. Write to satisfy the reader's ear as well as his intellect.
6. Let a little of your personality and good nature season your writing.

REFERENCES

Fowler HW, Fowler FG: *The King's English,* ed 3. Oxford, Oxford University Press, 1934.

Leacock S: *How to Write.* New York, Dodd, Mead & Co, Inc, 1943.

Quiller-Couch A: *On the Art of Writing.* New York, Capricorn Books, 1961.

Strunk W Jr, White EB: *The Elements of Style.* New York, The Macmillan Co, 1962.

III

Blunders and Blather:

The Pathology of Language

10

Faults of Word Choice

The truth, says an old proverb, is one, but error is many-headed. Though it would be quite impossible to catalog all the ways in which the technical writer can stray into ambiguity, inelegance or nonsense, I can at least show how and why, in actual practice, writers most often do stray. The ablest harbor pilot is the one with the most accurate knowledge of shoals and reefs, and clearest idea where not to take a ship.

In this chapter and the two which follow I have tried to classify common errors peculiar to medical writing, drawing most of my examples from actual published material. In a few instances I have improved on nature and made a blunder more glaring than it was. In many other cases I have had to correct one or more mistakes in a specimen so that they would not distract the reader from the mistake that I wanted to discuss.

Inexperience and poor judgment, the chief sources of trouble in writing, can both be cured by practice. In the act of putting his thoughts on paper the inexperienced writer is continually assailed by temptations to wander from his purpose of expressing himself clearly and logically. Convinced that plain English sounds unscientific, he translates *give* to *administer* and *stretch* to *elongation,* and recasts "The patient felt pain" as "The patient reported experiencing a sensatin of discomfort." Fearful that concise statements are unclear, he qualifies and elaborates them with superfluous adjectives, adverbs, prepositional phrases and other verbal clutter.

The unpracticed writer who feels that standard terminology and forthright syntax are dull and commonplace may try to enliven his writing with constructions reminiscent of pulp fiction at its worst. Mistaking simplicity of expression for baldness, he swells out his phrases with tasteless grandiloquence, and in laboring to avoid repetition creates a grotesque heterogeneity of word and idiom.

Another large class of language disorder results from ignorance or neglect of the principles of grammar and punctuation which were reviewed in Chapters 4 and 5. Many of those principles will be considered again here from the viewpoint of morbid anatomy. Few of the errors discussed in these final chapters occur in pure culture or flourish in isolation. That is, inaccuracy, inexactness, obscurity, inelegance and eccentricity all overlap broadly. I have not tried to analyze my specimens in detail, but have been content with stating the main objection to each. The faults discussed in the present chapter, various though they are in appearance, all consist in the wrong choice of a word or phrase.

SUBSTANDARD AND UNIDIOMATIC USAGE

*Just because the pain of biliary colic subsides abruptly does not mean that the stone has been expelled into the duodenum.

*At each contact with such a patient the clinician must try and foresee patterns of noncompliance, and take steps to prevent them.

*Some of these solutions can be used as is from the vial.

*The acquired form of the disease may well be contracted and the patient never know it, a subclinical-type process.

Just because . . . doesn't mean, try and, as is and the sense-blurring enclitic *-type* may pass in speech, but they are offensive in print. The writer who cannot expunge these colloquialisms from his formal style is in danger of being taken for an ignoramus or an illiterate. Fashions in formal usage come and go. Less objectionable, but still decidedly substandard, are such expressions as *later on* for *later, people* for *persons,* and *a couple* for *two.*

*Pain in the neck may be caused from irritation of the diaphragmatic pleura.

*Invasion of spirochetes into the eyes may lead to chorioretinitis, iritis and iridocyclitis.

*Normal Infant Delivered of a Woman with Cushing's Syndrome.

Each of these examples uses a preposition in an unidiomatic way. Pain is caused *by* irritation. Invasion *of* the eye *by* spirochetes may damage the uveal tract. An infant can be delivered *by* or *to* a woman, or a woman can be delivered *of* an infant. The variants quoted above are not English.

*Nausea and vomiting may occur because of the muscle-relaxing
   properties of diazoxide on the stomach.
*In second degree block the exercise response of the heart may be in-
   adequate though its function is not autonomous of sympathetic
   control.
*The results cannot be interpreted with confidence unless the second
   aspiration is made in the exact manner as the original.

In each case the writer has joined a connective to another word in a way
that violates English idiom. *Properties, autonomous* and *exact* cannot
legitimately figure in constructions like these. Diazoxide exerts a muscle-
relaxing *effect on* the stomach. The heart is not *free* (or *independent*) of
sympathetic control. The second aspiration must be made in the *same*
manner as the first.

Diagnose from, as in "The early stages of rheumatoid arthritis may be
difficult to diagnose from acute rheumatic fever," has the authority of
many eminent medical writers, including Osler, though in our day the
more usual expressions are *differentiate from* and *distinguish from.*

*Physicians and pharmacists can allay much unnecessary concern by
   warning patients of potential drug-induced urine dis-
   coloration.
*Atopy is the only reliable indication that a patient is in jeopardy of
   developing an anaphylactoid reaction.
*Hyperbaric oxygen is still an inconclusive technique of therapy.
*The ultrasonogram can help preclude a suspected extopic
   pregnancy.
*If the ovum is not fertilized the corpus luteum gradually de-
   generates and scarifies.
*It was this second body of data that led Kastner to hypothecate an
   antioxidant principle in the soil.
*Finally one of the nurses surprised the patient in the act of giving
   herself a factitious injection of insulin.

The errors here are malapropisms or, more formally, catachreses. In each
sentence a word has been wrongly substituted for another with a similar
sound or meaning. Physicians and pharmacists should be enjoined to
prevent concern, not merely *allay* it; one cannot allay something until it
has come into being. A person who is at risk, or in danger, of developing
an anaphylactoid reaction may be *in jeopardy of his life,* but the sentence quoted above is gibberish. The evidence in favor of hyperbaric
oxygen therapy may be inconclusive, but the technique itself is *unproved.*
Preclude means *prevent or render impossible,* not *rule out.* Scarification

is a surgical procedure (Greek *skariphos=stylus, lancet*); it does not mean *cicatrization* ("scarring"). *Hypothecate* is a legal term referring to a pledge or security; it does not mean *form* or *state a hypothesis*. *Surreptitious* injection of insulin may cause factitious (bogus, contrived) hypoglycemia, but the injection itselt cannot be called factitious if it has really taken place.

These blunders follow no pattern or principle, though most of them are created by false analogy with correct words or usages. Lapses like these will never be purged from the medical literature as long as writers and editors decline to serve an apprenticeship to truly competent and cultivated authors.

VERBAL INEXACTNESS

When a paper begins with an absurdity like "The rubella virus was first isolated by two different laboratories," who wants to read further? If the author gets away with so flagrant an abuse of language in his first sentence, what will he be up to by the last? Only one of the two "different" laboratories can have been first. The impossibility of being sure which one it was scarcely justifies the statement that they were both first. In technical writing there are no little white lies.

As the variety of errors in this class is unlimited, there is not much profit in an extensive survey. Let a few examples suffice.

> *The intercostal vessels and nerves pass in an intermuscular plane between each rib.

Though the old distinction, *between two, among more than two,* is nearly defunct, neither *between* nor *among* can take an object that is singular in both form and meaning. The intercostal vessels and nerves lie *between each pair of ribs, between the ribs,* or *beneath each rib*.

> *In fiscal 1975, every man, woman and child in the United States spent an average of $547 for health care.

Here we find a numerical datum expressed in the murky jargon of the lay press. *Average* is incompatible with *every man, woman and child*. One of them has to go, preferably the *every* phrase, which turns the statement into a statistical fiction.

> *Blood cultures should be repeated three times at 12- to 18-hour intervals before initiation of antibiotic therapy.

Since a procedure cannot be *repeated* until it has already been done at least once, a more suitable word here would be *done* or *performed*.

> *The 500 infected recruits at Fort Dix had no contact with swine; they gave the disease to each other.

Carelessness with universal words like *all, each, none* frequently produces nonsense, as it has done here. We might as well say that two barracudas ate each other.

> *The patient had had four to five prior episodes of pericarditis.

It is possible to have five to 10 episodes, or to have a condition for four to five years. But since an episode, unlike a year, is indivisible, there is no range of possibilities between four episodes and five. Replace *to* with *or*.

Many common usages in medicine are indefensibly inexact. We speak of a *reversal* of the albumin/globulin ratio when we mean only that the ratio is abnormal. We refer to *subclinical jaundice* as though jaundice could exist without being observed; we mean *subclinical hyperbilirubinemia.* We distinguish renal failure from *prerenal failure,* though it is not clear what is supposed to be failing in the latter. These and most of the other common verbal inaccuracies mentioned throughout the book are caprices of usage, which freely discards the literal or historical meaning of a word and substitutes an entirely different one in defiance of logic and common sense.

The following pairs of terms are often confused. The words in parentheses are meant to distinguish, not define.

accuracy (correctness)	precision (sharpness of focus)
congenital (from birth)	hereditary (inherited)
continual (repeated)	continuous (unbroken)
factitious (faked)	factitial (accidental)
ligature (tying)	suture (sewing)
occlusion (closing up)	stenosis (narrowing)
prevalence (extent)	incidence (attack rate)
sensitivity (few false negatives)	specificity (few false positives)

ARGOT

To the uninitiated, the typical physical examination record must read like a litany of lunacy borrowed from the pages of Rabelais or Lear: "The patient is oriented in three spheres . . . the grin is symmetrical . . . the tongue protrudes in the midline . . . .'' Expressions such as *gallbladder diet, tracheal toilet* and *light chains in the urine* are highly susceptible to misinterpretation by the nonphysician.

To object on these grounds to the use of argot in technical writing would be fatuous. For example, "Most deep-vein thrombi are clinically silent" is professional slang which every physician understands, even though it may be bewildering to a layman. In the same class is "The radiologist noted no joint mice but recommended sunset and tunnel views."

Some slang, however, should be reserved for informal conversation and not allowed to get into print. Avoid excessively crude and tasteless language borrowed from general slang.

> *The patient continued to look rocky.
> *The typical member of the Geritol set lives from one bowel movement to the next.

The objectionableness of such freedom in formal writing is so evident as to require no further discussion. The cultivated writer also avoids *better off, stay put, "Proteus* was the culprit" and "The differential diagnosis is not all that difficult."

Argot that is not plain in meaning to every English-speaking physician must be carefully kept out of printed matter that is expected to travel outside the United States. In this class may be placed *hard data, blood picture, garden-variety essential hypertension, split renal functions* and "The patient was covered with penicillin." Elliptical terms like "pars [interarticularis] defect" and "caput [succedaneum]," and vivid figures like "positive chandelier sign" are not necessarily in international use.

Even when an elliptical expression is perfectly plain it may violate editorial standards. For example, though "falciparum malaria" and "mg%" may seem respectable enough, they are actually shorthand for *"Plasmodium falciparum* malaria" and "mg/dl" or "mg/100 ml," and a strict and conscientious editor will insist on the fuller and more formal expressions. "The Weber lateralizes to the right" contains both an ellipsis (for *Weber's test*) and a jargon word, but the full expression represented by *lateralizes* is so cumbersome that most editors will accept the shorter form (while insisting on *Weber's test*).

"The patient is critical" nowadays means that he may not live; a century ago it would have suggested only that he might not pay. Here, too, we have an ellipsis (for *in critical condition*) of a kind extremely common in medical slang. The sinoatrial node is called simply *the sinus,* while *the node* invariably refers to the atrioventricular node. "The patient was fibrillating" will not get past an alert editor. *Poliovirus* is compact and intelligible, but *polio* for *poliomyelitis* is still slang. So are *acute* (for *short-term*) *therapy* and *acute* (for *sudden*) *release of thyroid hormone.* Even "The patient was begun on . . ." is slightly vulgar.

Carefully avoid argot that is inexact, lending itself to diverse interpretations or perhaps saying something false. The following sentences appeared in separate papers in a "symposium" on medical emergencies.

> Coma may be divided into four classes: supratentorial mass lesions, infratentorial mass or destructive lesions, metabolic-toxic encephalopathy and psychogenic "coma."
>
> Since the site of the major abnormality in these patients seems to be supratentorial, therapy should be directed toward the relief of anxiety.

In the first sentence *supratentorial* has its literal anatomic meaning; in the second it is slang for *mental, emotional,* or *psychogenic.* Though the nonphysician is generally a better judge than the physician of what is argot and what is not, in this case the editor could hardly have been expected to distinguish the two meanings of the word.

The reverse problem arises in "The electrocardiogram showed no acute changes and no changes from the previous tracing." Though this is acceptable medical writing, to an editor it will seem redundant unless he understands that the second use of *changes* is to be taken literally whereas the first means *signs, deviations from the normal.*

Another example of inexact argot appears in "The urine was negative for bile." The appearance of bile in the urine would be remarkable indeed. If we amend the sentence to read, "The urine was negative for bilirubin," it is still argot—*negative for* in this sense is certainly not standard English—but here the compression is not achieved at the expense of truth.

FIGURES OF SPEECH

In the last chapter, while discussing metaphor as a means of enhancing the appeal of medical writing, I hinted that rhetorical figures sometimes have dangerous side-effects. When metaphor, hyperbole and other such figures are introduced at the wrong places in technical writing they subtract from the precision and directness that the reader has a right to expect. A metaphor is not merely inexact; it is a deliberate falsehood. It is not true that the cephalic vein *plunges* into the supraclavicular fossa, that statistics can *drug* us into complacency, or that a diabetic is *brittle*. The medical writer would do well to take to heart Cicero's advice: "A metaphor ought always to be introduced with diffidence."

A number of medical metaphors might be rather strongly condemned if they were not so deeply entrenched. Thus, *distant* heart tones are muffled or indistinct but not really distant. *Rare* posterior cervical nodes are few in number, not rare. A *wide* pulse pressure is excessive, not wide. These and others like them will generally pass muster in formal writing.

However, metaphors and numerical data do not mix.

*The mortality of infants above 1000 gm declines rapidly.

Declines rapidly is at best a loose figure drawn from the shape of a curve on a graph, in which the *x* axis is fancifully taken to represent time ("rapidly") instead of weight. Though the meaning may be evident, the figure is better suited to the newspapers than to scientific writing.

*Alopecia areata may crop up independently or as part of the overall syphilitic syndrome.
*Finally the hyperuricemia crystallized as an episode of gross hematuria.
*The thoracic and cardiovascular surgeon may be still less at home below the navel.

Surely no comment is needed here.

An indolent writer may find that a metaphor is a handy way to avoid confronting an issue directly.

*Systemic hypotension may *spell* a reduction in circulating sympathetic amines.

Cause, result from, be a sign of? Leave such words to the tabloid writers, who have a license to imply more than they say, and say more than they know.

Whereas a metaphor calls something by a false name outright ("The liver is a factory"), a simile makes a comparison ("as dark as Coca-Cola"), or at least implies one ("stony induration"). A metaphor is pure embroidery, but because a simile can be taken literally it may serve to clarify an idea by making it more vivid and concrete. The usefulness of a simile in technical writing depends on its aptness and intelligibility.

Some comparisons are worse than useless. What is "the diameter of an egg''? In the first place an egg is not round, and in the second its dimensions are by no means fixed even if the reference is limited to hens' eggs. (For pertinent and amusing commentary on this topic see Holleb AI: Fruits, vegetables and cancer. *CA, A Cancer Journal for Clinicians* 25:112, 1975, and letters written in response to it, 25:278-279, 1975; also Hardy JW: Size of mammary lumps. *JAMA* 234:1321, 1975.) An American physician who compares the size of a lesion to that of a buckeye or a black-eyed pea might react with indignation if a foreign writer referred to the thickness of a banyan root or the diameter of a cricket ball.

A few medical comparisons that do not concern size are also ambiguous. *Tunnel vision,* when applied to one eye, means concentric field contraction with macular sparing, but as a description of binocular vision it means bitemporal hemianopia. The term *clay-colored stool* evidently refers to china clay and pipe clay. But because "clay" can be black, brown, yellow or red as well as white (fittingly enough, since all men are made of it), its color spectrum completely overlaps that of normal stool.

So-called shotty lymph nodes are neither as small nor as hard as any pieces of shot in modern use. In any event, the ubiquitous misspelling *shoddy,* which is becoming the rule even in journals of some prestige, has virtually robbed the figure of all significance. I do not propose to expunge *tunnel vision, clay-colored stool* and *shotty lymph nodes* from the physician's working vocabulary. I only urge that inventors of new similes exercise as much care as if they were coining formal technical terms.

There should be no need to present a formal case against hyperbole in medical writing. Medicine may not be an exact science but its practitioners are expected to be exact at least in recording dimensions and other numerical facts. In the last chapter I justified one or two jesting exaggerations on the grounds that they enlivened a narrative or highlighted a major point. But hyperbole cannot be tolerated in what purports to be a statement of fact.

    *Ampicillin rash sometimes looks more like rubella than rubella itself.

    *After incision the lesion may continue discharging pus by the bucket for several days.

On the other hand, "studied neglect" (adapted no doubt from Disraeli's "policy of masterly inactivity") is firmly established in medical parlance, and has a clear and constant meaning. Strictly speaking it is not a hyperbole but an oxymoron.

Presumably the author who writes of "inadvertent collapse of a valve leaflet'' does not realize what he is saying. *Inadvertent* means not *accidental* or *catastrophic* but *without attention or awareness.* Can a valve leaflet be attentive to or aware of its own collapse? Anthropomorphism, endowing inanimate things with human characters and qualities, is a universal practice, and by no means wholly objectionable even in technical writing. (See Schoenfeld R: This article explains. . . . *Proc Roy Austral Chem Inst* 42:129-130, 1975.) In the following examples, however, the writers have strayed beyond the bounds of reason.

> *A strategically placed goiter can cause tracheal compression or displacement, or both.
> *With smaller degrees of vasoconstriction the Korotkoff sounds underestimate the systolic pressure and overestimate the diastolic pressure.
> *The rate of absorption of aqueous humor exactly balances its rate of manufacture.

Some critics have objected to the frequent use of *demonstrate, display, disclose, exhibit* and *reveal* in clinical reportage. As these words inject both color and variety, it seems a shame to forbid them absolutely. Common sense should protect the writer against extremes like the following.

> *The dorsum of the foot reveals a thinner and more sensitive skin than the sole.

VERBAL EQUIVOCATION

When a word has more than one meaning, some clue must accompany it so that the reader can choose the intended meaning at once. A *fundus* may be either uterine or optic, a *steroid* either adrenocortical or anabolic. "The cord" is spinal to a neurologist, umbilical to an obstetrician, spermatic to a urologist.

> *The catheter tip was located in the left atrium.
> *Circulating erythrocytes are destroyed during the normal aging process.
> *Petit mal seizures may be abolished by reduction of cellular pH.

Locate, which crouches irresolutely on the fence between good English and hyperurbanism, is best avoided in medical writing. In the above example, *was located* could mean either *was placed, was found,* or simply *was.* In the second sentence *aging* is at least slightly ambiguous.

In the third, *abolish* could mean either stopping an individual seizure or controlling the seizure disorder.

Sometimes through carelessness a writer leaves the reader in doubt as to what part of speech a word is meant to be. Does "the importance of patient demonstration" mean demonstration *with patience* or *to patients*?

Special care is needed with certain words denoting comparison or change. An *improvement in frequency* means a decrease if the patient has cystitis but just the opposite if his complaint is impotence. The greater curvature of the stomach has a longer radius than the lesser curvature, besides describing a longer arc. But when the cornea is said to have a greater curvature than the surrounding sclera, a shorter radius of curvature is meant. An "increased carrying angle" at the elbow should not be recorded as 150° but as 30° (that is, 180°-150°), since what has increased is not the angle between arm and forearm but the divergence from a straight line.

REDUNDANCY

Some degree of redundancy is unavoidable in our language. When we say "*Insert* the speculum gently *in* the nostril" we repeat the *in* because *sert* without the prefix is not a word. In *prognathous jaw* we are compelled to restate the idea of *jaw* already inherent in *prognathous* (from Greek *gnathos = jaw*), since *prognathism* refers to the condition but not to the jaw itself, and *prominent* or *protruding jaw* would not be specific enough.

Clearly distinct from such inescapable repetitions of morpheme or idea is the sentence which contains an entirely superfluous word or phrase. For example, a negligent writer may insert a word twice in a long sentence. The commonest victim of this syntactic stuttering is the conjunction *that*.

> *It is becoming apparent that if the use of amphetamines in obesity is not sharply retrenched by the medical profession that the federal watchdogs will do it for us.

A sentence with a subjunctive verb sometimes parades a whole series of redundant auxiliary verbs.

> *On exploration the surgeon may discover that the lesion may be quite otherwise than he may have suspected.

Too common in technical writing is the construction in which one word or phrase exactly echoes another, which often stands immediately adjacent: *traumatic injury, continued daily re-evaluation.* A modifier is pleonastic when its meaning is implicit in its headword: *female ovary, human children, reopen again, retract back.*

>   *The written examination is administered *twice annually* every spring and fall at various centers distributed *geographically* around the country.

In each of the following sentences one or the other of the italicized parts may stand, but not both.

>   **The reason for* this stoppage is not *due to* the normal limit of motion of the joint.
>   **With the exception of the index case* all *other* patients recovered in less than a week.

Such as . . . and so forth is usually an improper combination. A phrase beginning *such as* is expected to sketch the limits of a class by giving examples of its members. Until the class stands clearly delineated it is unfair to the reader to say "and *so* forth," "and the *like*," "and others of the *same* kind." Once the class has been defined it is pointless to mention other members in such vague terms. There is no objection, however, to a concluding phrase in which the focus is sharpened: "such as the skin, the central nervous system *and other ectodermal derivatives.*"

VERBS

Carefully observe the limitations placed by formal usage on the construction of predicates (see Chapter 4). In each of the following sentences the complement does not fit the verb.

>   *This technique has proved 98% effective in *enabling* selection of the proper antibiotic. BETTER: *guiding, directing, making possible*
>   *The patient's family physician could not *convince* him to undergo arteriography. BETTER: *persuade*
>   *The wound edges may be *imbedded* with dirt. BETTER: Dirt may be imbedded in the wound edges.

It is not possible to convert every intransitive verb to a transitive one simply by supplying it with an object. Avoid substandard and unidiomatic usages like the following.

*Slimming down to ideal weight often *reverts* serum triglycerides to normal. BETTER: *restores*

*Saline irrigation alone may suffice to *emerge* the stone into the ampulla. BETTER: *expel*

The fabrication of a new verb by back-formation from a noun or other part of speech has been a common practice in English for centuries. It is perfectly legitimate to form the verb *to ligate* from *ligation.* The back-formation is concise and specific, and it is only a matter of chance that the noun *ligation* entered English from Latin by way of French before we had a corresponding verb.

Some back-formations, however, are superfluous. In Chapter 2 I mentioned *to replete* as a vulgar rival of *to replenish.* Similarly, *orientate,* from *orientation,* is an unneeded variant of *orient,* and *fixate,* from *fixation,* is no improvement on *fix.*

Back-formations generally wear some kind of verbal suffix, most often *-ate* from the Latin participle ending *-atum* or the noun ending *-atio.* Others derived from Latin stems have remnants of irregular participle forms (*torse,* from *torsion; percuss,* from *percussion; infarct,* from *infarction*). Many back-formations from Greek nouns end in *-ose,* adapted from *-osis* (*diagnose, necrose*).

The decision whether to use a back-formation should be based on three considerations: Is there already a simpler verb from the same stem? Is there a suitable verb from a different stem? Is the succinctness of the new verb outweighed by its irregularity or uncouthness? Verbs that fail the last test include *to liaise* (originally American military cant, from *liaison*), *to seize* (= to have a seizure) and *to diaphorese.*

Another common and ancient way of forming a new verb is to use a noun as a verb without changing it at all. Many of Shakespeare's happiest inventions are nouns that have been *verbed.* Despite his example ("it out-herods Herod") and that of such modern words as *lynch* and *boycott,* technical verbs made from proper names (to Foley, to Kocher) are usually slangy and should be kept out of print. Here again the conscientious writer will abstain from innovation when a suitable verb form is already available. (See Gode A: Just words, *JAMA* 190:508, 1964 and Schoenfeld R: To reflux or not to reflux? *Proc Roy Austral Chem Inst* 41:223-224, 1974.)

MODIFIERS

I have stated elsewhere that the principal tools of exposition are nouns and verbs. Adjectives and adverbs are second-string words, useful chiefly to clarify and distinguish. A modifier should never be used unless it is both exact and indispensable. Instead of adding anything, a superfluous adjective or adverb subtracts and distracts.

Do not count on an adjective to correct the damage done by the poor choice of a noun, or expect an adverb to redeem a weak or inappropriate verb. Choose strong, specific nouns and verbs in the first place and you will be in little danger of abusing or overworking modifiers.

In each of the following phrases an adjective that normally distinguishes a part has been illegitimately attributed to the whole.

*posterior skull
*spasm of the left neck and shoulder
*fracture of the distal radius
*dermatitis of the upper feet

Though this conventional shorthand is widely understood, it is shorthand all the same. What is meant is the posterior *part* of the skull, spasm of the left *side* of the neck, the distal *end* of the radius, the upper *surfaces* of the feet. Many such expressions bear the stamp of long and extensive usage (*proximal tubule, left heart failure*), but they all stretch the language out of shape, and careful writers and editors avoid them. (See Hussey HH: Medical jargon. *JAMA* 235:1149, 1976.)

A variant of this practice results in such phrases as *a severe arthritic, and acute schizophrenic* and *a mild diabetic,* where adjectives originally and properly applied to diseases have been somewhat inaccurately carried over to sufferers from those diseases. The injury done to language by these aberrations would be small were it not that some adjectives, including the three in my examples, have different meanings when applied to persons than when applied to diseases. Of course, if your arthritic is stern, your schizophrenic shrewd, and your diabetic kind and gentle, you may use such terms with impunity.

A superfluous adjective is often found in a statement about paired organs.

*Unilateral absence of the testis may be more crippling psycho-
   logically than sterility.
*Excretory urography demonstrated bilaterally small kidneys.

In each case a cumbersome modifier has been tacked onto a word that is perfectly clear as it stands. It is obvious that when one refers to a paired organ in the singular (*the testis*) he means only one, and when he uses the plural (*kidneys*) he means both. (See Arnold HL: Precision in description. *JAMA* 235:2286, 1976.)

More, most, less and *least* fall victim to many abuses. They are often found qualifying or comparing absolute terms, as in the following examples.

> *The discussant felt that the slides showed a more granulomatous process.
> *The procedure is less atraumatic but yields 60% improvement in accuracy.

In the first sentence the meaning is "granulomatous rather than something else" and, in the second, "more traumatic." Since *atraumatic* means literally *without injury* it is an absolute term. A few words formed with the Greek prefix *a-*, however, are not absolute in common parlance (*anemia*, for example) and can be compared. Similarly, many English adjectives which were originally absolute now have a relative connotation in speech, but these should probably not be compared or qualified in technical writing. Thus, *very minimal, less essential, relatively painless, more preliminary* and *least appreciable* are all mismatches.

A numerical comparison must be worded accurately.

> *Hyperkinetic children were five times *more likely than* normal children to have been born prematurely. BETTER: *as likely as*

Negative qualities must be compared with great caution. It is proper to say that one figure is lower than another, or one patient younger than another, but it is absolute nonsense to say "twice as low" or "twice as young." The following statements are bad English and worse arithmetic.

> *In nonsmokers the risk is six times lower.
> *In patients over 40 undergoing elective inguinal herniorrhaphy, low-dose heparin prophylaxis led to a sevenfold reduction in the incidence of deep-vein thrombosis.
> *One cup of decaffeinated coffee contains thirty times less caffeine than a cup of regular coffee.

Careful users of English preserve a sharp distinction between *less,* referring to a singular aggregate noun (*weight, medication, irrigant*) and *fewer,* referring to a plural noun (*seizures, injections, ml*). *Less calories* is advertiser's cant, not standard English. *Lesser* of course refers to size (*lesser peritoneal cavity*), not number. *Better* compares neither size nor number: *more* (not *better*) *than 100,000 colonies/cu mm; a diameter greater* (not *better*) *than 20 cm.*

Multiple should be reserved for things that are truly multiple (consisting of several parts) and not used as a fancy synonym for *many.*

*The umbilical ring may be dilated by ascites or multiple pregnan-
cies. (Triplets, or three pregnancies?)

Do not let adjectival prefixes stand alone like free morphemes.

*The patient then complained of substernal pain and had a semi
emesis.
*The shoulder had already been vigorously manipulated by a
pseudo osteopath.

Semi-, pseudo- and multi- are prefixes, not words, though there is no
fixed rule as to whether they should be fused with a stem or separated by
a hyphen. In forming an adjective with -like, be sure to put the suffix on
the right word: swine-influenza-like, not swine-like influenza.

Some authorities object to the use of increased, elevated, reduced and
diminished in the description of physical signs or laboratory test results
when the basis for comparison is an absolute standard, as in "Ausculta-
tion revealed diminished breath sounds over the right lung base." This
seems unduly strict. The meaning can hardly be mistaken, and the
avoidance of these common and useful words forces longer and more
cumbersome expressions on both writer and reader: "The breath sounds
are fainter than would be expected over the right lung base."

Medical writers lean rather heavily on a group of excessively vague and
noncommittal adjectives, which weaken and obscure rather than strength-
en and clarify. The typical physician would be at least slightly annoyed if
a nurse answered his inquiry about a patient's blood pressure with the
observation that it was "normal." Similarly, the medical writer should
not call anything normal when the reader has a right to determine for
himself whether it is normal or not.

Normal should never be stuck in as a hasty generalization when a
fuller and more precise statement is called for. Though it is generally
proper in a published case report to describe the ocular movements or
the consistency of the prostate as normal, it would scarcely be permissible, in a paper on pulmonary disease, to assert simply that "the
findings in the chest were normal."

Normal is seldom the right word to describe the result of a qualitative
test or of the attempt to find or elicit a sign. A test result is best reported as positive, negative or inconclusive. Even these terms are sometimes equivocal.

*A negative gastric aspiration is no assurance that the end of the
tube is not in the stomach.

*The patient reacted negatively to noxious stimuli.

"The patient *demonstrated a negative response* to dinitrochlorobenzene" is an elaborate and misleadingly oblique way of saying that nothing whatever happened. A sign is either present or absent. It is nonsense to say, "The Babinski reflex is normal." Either the *patient* is normal, in which case the Babinski reflex is not elicited (that is, is *absent*), or the reflex is present, in which case the patient is certainly not normal.

Using a farfetched synonym for *normal* ("The Romberg is intact," "The deep tendon reflexes are physiologic," "The abdomen was benign") does nothing to mitigate these faults. If *normal* invites the reader's skepticism, qualifying the word with an equally insipid adverb only seems to deepen the intrigue. *Grossly normal* may be translated as "apparently normal to the careless examiner." *Essentially normal* (like *noncontributory)* implies a private judgment or reservation by the writer.

The objections to the excessive and indiscriminate use of *somewhat, moderate, massive, gross* and *dramatic* are obvious. *Marked* often appears in contexts that belie its literal meaning ("Occasionally a tracheostomy is indicated if there has been marked inhalation of smoke"), and is still more often wholly adventitious ("Transverse scans showed enlargement of both kidneys, more marked on the left"). Probably a gallicism, it seems to have been a favorite adjective of medical writers for decades. Three of the nine examples of its use given in the *Oxford English Dictionary* are from medical works, the first dated 1797. (See Girone JA: Further elucidation of medical jargon. *NEJM* 286:382, 1972 and Hussey HH: Fashionable and objectionably fashionable. *JAMA* 236:1051, 1976.)

When an adjective has two forms, one ending in -*ic* and the other in -*ical*, the shorter is usually preferred. Exceptions fall into three classes.

1. The longer form is required when the -*ic*- is part of the stem: *apical, cortical.* (Shorter forms of these words are entirely improper.)

2. The longer form may have a different meaning: *historical* = *pertaining to history; historic* = *famous, noteworthy.*

3. The longer form may be preferred as a point of usage: *atypical, chemical, classical, clinical, hysterical, logical, mathematical, methodical, optical, pharmaceutical, spherical, statistical, surgical, theoretical, typical.* Shorter forms of these words vary from illicit to merely eccentric.

An adverb whose meaning is logically restricted to human activity should not modify a whole clause or sentence as in these examples.

*Thankfully these lesions almost always regress without treatment.

> *The patient is now receiving furosemide, which hopefully will
> correct the steroid-induced retention of water and mineral.

In the first sentence *fortunately* might be substituted for the irrational
adverb, but the second needs more drastic revision, since in English the
writer's hopes cannot properly be announced by any adverb whatever.
Perhaps this deficiency of our language helps to explain the popularity of
hopefully, whose use as a sentence adverb may have arisen by analogy
with German *hoffentlich.* In just a few years this curious solecism has
spread across the English-speaking world and become entrenched in the
diction of even the most perspicuous writers. (See Arnold HL: Some
hope remains. *JAMA* 234:383, 1975 and Southgate MT: A rococo report.
JAMA 237:1362, 1977.) Probably in time *hopefully* will be as respectable
as the equally silly sentence adverbs *doubtless* and *ironically.*

Another practice that may be related to a German usage is that of
forming rough-and-ready adverbs by adding the suffix *-wise* to nouns
(lungwise, electrolytewise) and adjectives *(pulmonarywise, hepaticwise).*
Similar adverbs are found in German and Scandinavian languages (cf.
German *tropfenweise = dropwise;* Swedish *delvis = partly),* but these languages do not form new words on these models as freely as does English.
Though *otherwise* and *likewise* have earned their patents of nobility,
"The functional deficit percentagewise is unchanged" is plebeian and
tasteless. (See Schoenfeld R: That's the way she crumbles, language-wise.
Proc Roy Austral Chem Inst 43:12-13, 1976.) Adverbs formed with
-ward (plantarward, rectumward) are less common but not more elegant.

The following sentences contain examples of an aberrant use of adverbs too frequently found in technical papers.

> *On the first occasion ampicillin was generically unobtainable.
> *The second heart sound is physiologically split.
> *The tonsils are surgically absent.
> *Each subject gave a detailed medical and surgical history and was
> examined physically.
> *Microscopically there was no major abnormality in the valve ring.
> *The patient finds it painfully impossible to stand on tiptoe.

In the first sentence the writer has made *generically unobtainable* the
equivalent of *not generally obtainable,* which itself forces the adverb into
an unidiomatic role. In the fourth sentence *examined physically* is offered as the equivalent of *subjected to physical examination.* The last
sentence is doubletalk. The writer's patient may find it painful to stand
on tiptoe, or he may find it impossible, but he cannot have it both ways.
Creating a jury-rigged surrogate for an adverbial phrase by adding *-ly* or

-*ally* to an adjective will often, as in these cases, distort meaning completely. "Men demonstrate no measurable superiority to women in intelligence" cannot be translated into "Men are immeasurably superior to women in intelligence."

Though, as noted in Chapter 5, the distinction between adjective and adverb is not always clear-cut, certain uses can be confidently labeled substandard and unidiomatic.

> *The glomus tumor is exquisitely painful, quite disproportionate [disproportionately] to its size.
> *The flaps are constructed such [so] that the anterior one cushions the end of the bone.
> *Silver sulfadiazine can ber used on exposed burns similar to [like] mafenide.

In the first two examples an adjective usurps the role of an adverb; in the third, of a preposition.

CONNECTIVES

In Chapter 5 I mentioned that some prepositions in common use began life as adjectives or participles: *prior to, depending on, including.* Many of these are so firmly established as connectives that their use causes no confusion. Indeed, a few (*during, notwithstanding*) are now pure prepositions. But some others still look like dangling modifiers to language purists and other finicky readers. Certainly there are cases in which these fledgling connectives do threaten both clarity and readability.

Due to can safely be used as a preposition most of the time, but on occasion may give rise to ambiguity. *Due* is still very much an adjective; its role is purely adjectival in "The graft was handled with all the care due to a tissue whose viability was already in doubt."

Based on probably owes much of its popularity to the feeling that it is shorthand for *on the basis of,* which is itself usually an inflated and pompous version of *as* or some other simple connective. (Thus, "They were treated as outpatients" becomes "They were treated on an outpatient basis.") But *based,* like *due,* is still an adjective (participle) in good standing, and on that account *based on* phrases are frequently awkward, though not always as equivocal as the following examples.

> *Dr. Rootens refutes erroneous views on aspirin sensitivity based on experience with private patients.
> *Verrucae respond to cryosurgery based not only on type but also on location.

   *The patient changed the therapeutic plan based on an irrational
      idea.

Sometimes a *based on* phrase is the reader's only clue that a statement is
an estimate or hypothesis rather than a fact.

   *Approximately 100,000 children with sickle-cell disease are born
      annually in Africa's sickle-cell belt based on the gene frequency
      and the birth rate.

Following for *after*, and *previous to* for *before*, are usually
clear enough but they detract slightly from the precision and vigor of
writing. Like them, the Latin words *per* and *via* inject a certain taint of
jargon into formal prose. *Per* is seldom appropriate except in units of
measure, and even then it is usually represented by a virgule (*mg/dl*) and
not written. *Per Foley, per vein* and the like are argot. If used at all, *via*
should preserve its correct and purely physical sense, *by way of,* as in
"via the periarticular anastomoses." The following is illiterate.

   *The ulcer gradually healed via astringent soaks, topical enzymes
      and gentamicin.

In re and *as per* are legalese, best left entirely out of medical writing.
   The use of *like* as a conjunction, in place of *as* and *as if*, though
deeply entrenched in speech, is still opposed by purists and eschewed by
the best writers.

   *These abnormal cells look like they have had a bite taken out of
      them.
   *He reacted to hyperventilation today just like he did before.

The substitution of *plus* for *and* or *besides*, except in mathematical expressions, is a vulgar philistinism.

   *Plus its muscular and cutaneous branches, the musculocutaneous
      nerve gives off a communicating branch on the dorsum of the
      foot to the sural nerve.

11

Faults of Syntax

The archetype of all syntactic errors is the anacoluthon, a change of horses in the middle of a sentence. The term denotes a complete breakdown of grammatical continuity, not just a shift of theme or viewpoint. Such lapses are abundant in dictated material, as anyone knows who reads his own dictations before signing them.

> *If there is a relationship between maternal coffee intake and the occurrence of apnea in the premature neonate, the assumption that the mother's drinking of coffee (or other methylxanthine-containing beverages) during labor to increase the amount of transplacentally acquired caffeine and therefore ameliorate or prevent the occurrence of apnea seems valid.
>
> *The observation that a nearly normal concentration of immunoreactive glucagon (IRG) was found in gastrointestinal tissues of depancreatized rats which had secreted a normal amount of IRG during insulin treatment and excessive amounts during insulin deprivation, suggesting that the gut is capable not only of secreting IRG but of storing it.

The authors of these overlong and unduly intricate sentences were probably so far from their points of origin when they finished that they forgot where they were going. Though anacoluthia is a constant feature of informal and even formal speech, its appearance in print usually bears witness to a conspiracy of carelessness between writer and editor. Occasionally, however, engrafting a parenthetical idea may lend both clarity

193

and compactness, even though technically it produces an anacoluthon: "He knows none better, that fried foods always cause a recurrence of his pain."

PLURAL CONSTRUCTIONS

Like most languages, English has many "illogical" usages involving plurals. We are not concerned here with established idioms like "the bag of waters" and "on all fours" but with the choice of a plural construction when a singular one would be clearer and more natural.

*The spinal fluid may contain large *quantities* of lead.
*The pupil dilated well with *mydriatics,* and the eye healed completely after treatment with *antibiotics* and padding.
*Radiographic studies showed degenerative changes in the thoracic and lumbar *spines.*
*Convalescent serum contained no *antibodies* to rubella virus.

Each example replaces an expected singular with an irrational plural. In the following sentences shifts from singular to plural or vice-versa emphasize the inappropriateness of the plural forms.

*Cervical spine injury was most likely to occur to *a linebacker or a defensive halfback* when *they* tackled the ball-carrier.
*In 1952 Zoll demonstrated that *the arrested heart* in *patients* with Adams-Stokes seizures could be sustained by intrathoracic pacing.
**Iodides* will retard the release of stored thyroid hormones. *This* can be administered as Lugol's solution or as sodium iodide.
*Over 50% of *patients* with hypertension caused by renal artery stenosis have *an abdominal bruit.*

ILL-ADVISED ELLIPSIS

I have observed elsewhere that overzealous efforts to achieve succinctness can pare a sentence too near the quick. A sentence can stand on one leg if you take the trouble to balance it properly, but if you cut off both legs no amount of effort can keep it upright. Even when it interrupts grammatical continuity a deliberate ellipsis may pass muster if it leaves the meaning intact: "In the strictest sense it is incorrect to speak of dominant or recessive genes, but only of dominant or recessive effects." But something essential for clarity has been left out of each of the following sentences, with results ranging from awkwardness to obscurity.

*Unlike the Insecta, the thorax and abdomen in ticks are fused.
*A common problem is to distinguish between an enlarged spleen and left kidney. (*And the left kidney,* or *and an enlarged left kidney?*)
*The Epstein-Barr antibody, where available, may be of great help in diagnosis.
*The position of the needle is then changed and is passed upward along the axis of the sacral canal for about 3 cm.
*Whenever feasible, a tracheostomy should be avoided.
*Although asymptomatic in some, many patients have alternating diarrhea and constipation.
*Special care via the intravenous route is warranted.
*Usually bilateral, occasionally one palpebral fissure is much wider than the other.
*Although originally reported that propranolol reduced the morality of acute myocardial infarction, these findings have since been refuted.

Some of these sentences might with equal propriety be offered as specimens of simple anacoluthia or dangling modifier.

The following are examples of a variation known as syllepsis, in which a word is forced to serve in two different senses at once.

*An increase in the size and firmness of the nodes of Hodgkin's disease signals recurring activity of the disease and further therapy. (*Signals* means both *gives evidence of* and *shows the need for.*)
*Marijuana reduces but does not totally alleviate intraocular pressure in glaucoma. (*Pressure* means both an absolute measurement and an abnormally high tension.)

NONPARALLELISM

Inconsistency or lack of parallelism in thought and idea—mingling fractions and decimals, apples and oranges—is seldom a danger for the author who is in full command of his subject. Grammatical inconsistency, though a more superficial and mechanical fault, is far commoner. A shift in grammatical construction where parallelism is expected can throw the reader off the track, sometimes without his awareness.

*There are regional differences both in the incidence [of urolithiasis] and [in the] type of kidney stone found. (Each ellipsis destroys a parallel.)

>*Arrhythmias due to catecholamine excess may occur during induc-
> tion of anesthesia, strenuous excercise and pheo-
> chromocytoma.
>*There are conflicting reports on a relationship between those drink-
> ing several cups of coffee daily and increased risk of heart
> attack.
>*Erysipelas is seldom seen nowadays either in the wards or in out-
> patients.
>*It is less painful to infiltrate both wound edges from proximal to
> distal *instead of going* [*than to go*] down one side and up the
> other.

In the first two examples parallelism can be restored by supplying missing words; in the third, by excising a surplus one (*those*). A frequent
cause of nonparallelism is a shift from active to passive voice.

>*While increased methemalbumin *is reported* by some authors to be
> diagnostic of hemorrhagic pancreatitis, others *feel* that it is
> nonspecific.
>*Rather than *set* up the appropriate studies, the drug *was with-
> drawn.*
>*The instrument is easily fabricated from available materials, [is]
> simple to handle, and avoids the discomfort that often follows
> prolonged use of standard pickups.

The last specimen exemplifies both ellipsis and voice shift as causes of
nonparallelism.

A change of tense disturbs the balance less violently but is still poor
composition.

>*Allgood and Putz *have shown* that flow rate is nearly constant
> when the pressure remains in the optimal range, but Gammard
> *reports* significant variations even under these circumstances.

LOOSE REFERENCE

Under this heading we might include many cases of sloppy syntax, but
we are chiefly interested here in the pronoun without an immediately
obviously antecedent.

>*This baby was admitted at 3:00 a.m. with a presumptive diagnosis
> of acute appendicitis. Probably it has already ruptured by
> then.

Though an instant's reflection shows that what had ruptured was the appendix, not the baby, it is the writer's duty to spare his reader that instant's reflection.

*The patient's father had asked the physician to see him but he felt that he would rather not discuss his case with him in detail.

This would probably be clear enough in conversation, but the writer is held to a much stricter standard of intelligibility than the speaker. A simple calculation shows that this sentence admits to no fewer than 144 possible interpretations, so that it is indeed grossly ambiguous.

*Intense arterial spasm may result from injection into its lumen.
*Paronychia may become chronic and produce recurrent cellulitis. These require excision of the involved tissue proximal to the nail fold.

In the first example the antecedent of *its* has moved and left no forwarding address, the writer apparently having forgotten that he had replaced the expected subjective genitive, *of an artery,* with an adjective. The writer of the second descends into incoherence by pointlessly shifting to the plural. Both violate the general rule that a pronoun should not be used unless its antecedent has *gone before* (Latin *antecedens = going before*) and survives in the reader's memory vividly enough to be recalled instantly.

LAX COORDINATION AND SUBORDINATION

The chief means at the writer's disposal for showing the relation between two clauses is the conjunction. Many writers undervalue conjunctions, choosing them almost haphazardly and failing to exploit to the full their power of uniting, dividing and organizing ideas. The aimless pairing of sentences with *and,* a device imported from novelese, weakens the semantic coherence of a paragraph.

*Many important structures lie beneath the glutus maximus, and to understand them the piriformis muscle may be used as a guide.
*Trimethoprim-sulfamethoxazole is highly effective in urinary tract infections and probably should not be used as a first-choice drug.

In the second example the simple coordination of two ideas with *and* throws away the opportunity to delineate their exact relation. *But* would be an improvement. Better still, a brief clause could be added to explain why a highly effective drug should not be used as a first choice.

> *Eleven months ago Dr. Palfrey performed an islet-cell transplant and the patient's daily insulin requirement dropped from 80 to 30 units.

Here again *and*, the feeblest of all conjunctions, loosely strings together two events whose temporal sequence, at least, deserves to be made clear. The practice of implying temporal and even causal relationships with *and* in technical writing is pernicious and deplorable.

> *Menorrhagia refers to totally irregular menses, prolonged in duration but not excessive in amount, *although* at times there may be only spotting.
> *Prophylactic administration of antibiotics should not be considered unless clinical or bacteriologic evidence of infection is found, *but* an aggressive therapeutic plan should be followed because the mortality rate of acute pancreatitis is as high as 40%.

In each of these examples the italicized word makes a concession that does not aptly reflect the relationship between the ideas. The real fault in each case is that matter for two sentences has been carelessly crammed into one.

Be sure that a concessive conjunction (*though, although*) introduces the concession and not the main statement.

> *Although viruses are suspected as the cause of these exanthems, failure to transmit them to laboratory animals other than monkeys has hindered definitive investigation.

Logic demands that *although* precede *failure to transmit*, while rhetoric gently urges that the clauses be reversed.

> BETTER: Although failure to transmit these exanthems to laboratory animals other than monkeys has hindered definitive investigation, viruses are suspected as the cause.

> *Pregnant diabetics should receive the vaccine because it will not harm the fetus.

We expect *because* to introduce a reason. Obviously the mere safety of a drug is never the reason for giving it. What is meant here is that a pregnant diabetic *may* receive the vaccine, *since* it will not harm the fetus.

*I have found neither circumstantial nor objective evidence to
support the theory of Niemeyer et al.

Circumstantial and objective evidence are not mutually exclusive; some would say that they overlap almost completely. Though the simple disjunctives *or* and *nor* may be used in this loose fashion, the correlatives *either . . . or* and *neither . . . nor* may not.

MISPLACED AND DISJOINTED PHRASES

The analysis of a confusing sentence often shows that although all needed words are present they have been arranged in helter-skelter sequence. It is amazing how much of this we can get away with in speech: "He ran off with the man who works at the pickle factory's wife." A particularly common source of trouble in writing is a **misplaced phrase** which stands too far from what it modifies or too close to what it does not modify.

*Microscopic inspection of the stools showed fat globules stained
with Sudan III.
*As a result of pregame taping we have noticed no significant change
in frequency and severity of ankle injuries.

The first sentence is no doubt true as it stands, but the last four words logically belong closer to *stools*. In their present position they suggest that the patient has been ingesting Sudan III. In the second example, *as a result of pregame taping* belongs at the end of the sentence, closer to *no significant change* than to *we have noticed*.

Most misplaced phrases are not equivocal but only awkward.

*Take Bayer aspirin for the fastest most gentle to the stomach
relief you can get from pain.

Though there is no ambiguity here, the word order is anomalous enough to give one a headache. Of nineteen examples of conspicuously clumsy writing quoted by Hussey, ten contain misplaced phrases. (Hussey HH: Unfelicitous medical writing. *JAMA* 238:897, 1975.)

In a **suspended construction** the reader is required to hang onto one half of a phrase while searching through the rest of the sentence for the other half.

*The lingual nerve passes downward deep to the external and on the
surface of the internal pterygoid muscle.
*The absorption into and distribution of penicillin in the central
nervous system leaves much to be desired.

Getting the separated words together again is well within the capacity of
the intelligent reader, but it is a nuisance all the same. Moreover, it often
prompts a hasty and inattentive scanning of the words between. Always
resist the temptation to write a suspended construction when more than
three or four words must intervene. A better word order can invariably
be found. Instead of "in the same manner as, though to a lesser degree
than, the Krebs cycle," write as you would speak: "in the same manner
as the Krebs cycle, though to a lesser degree." Even a short suspension
of continuity may endanger grammatical parallelism, as in "the most
important and certainly one of the largest ganglia." The suspended
phrase, *the most important . . . ,* can logically be completed only by a
singular noun (*ganglion*). Here again a simple rearrangement of the
words effects a cure: "the most important ganglion, and certainly one of
the largest."

*The child is constantly reminded to keep his head straight under a
drill, as opposed to an automatic response, program.
*Both edematous and hemorrhagic pancreatitis produce colloid,
electrolyte and fluid imbalance because of peripancreatic
edema.
*Histologic examination revealed no significant renal lesions, de-
generative changes in liver cells, and acute diffuse alveolar
damage.

These are cases of **phrasal miscue.** The reader, never suspecting that he is
on the wrong tack, goes blithely and confidently forward until he is up
to his neck in quicksand. In the first and second sentences, suspended
constructions are responsible for most of the trouble. The first gives us
the chilling impression that the physical therapist is about to treat
psychomotor retardation with a burrhole in the cranium. In the second
we initially take *colloid* for a noun instead of an adjective. In the third
we expect *no* to modify all three pathologic changes mentioned, and do
not see our error (which is really not ours but the writer's) until we have
nearly finished the sentence.

Here is another sentence in which negative and positive ideas have
been shuffled out of the logical order.

*This product differs from the USP ointment in that it contains the same proportion of zinc oxide as the USP ointment [utter non-sense so far] but has a different base, containing benzoinated petrolatum and white wax instead of liquid petrolatum and white ointment.

In a **jumbled phrase** the words stand in an order that belies their proper and logical relation. The difference between *a distilled flask of water* and *a flask of distilled water* goes deeper than syntax; the first is a downright absurdity. Equally senseless are the italicized phrases in the following specimens.

> *These findings are incompatible with *the presence of probable pericardial effusion.*
> **A shattered fragment of the left ischiopubic ramus* penetrated the rectum.
> *At laparotomy she was found to have *a segment of necrotic small bowel.*

Avoiding such baroque ensembles demands unfaltering attention to the business of composition. Note that many phrases on the same model are perfectly acceptable either way: *administration of prophylactic antibiotics* does not differ substantially from *prophylactic administration of antibiotics.*

AMPHIBOLY

When a construction admits of two or more interpretations, and nothing but outside information can resolve the dilemma, the fault is known as amphiboly. This is to be distinguished from verbal equivocation (see Chapter 10), in which the sense or bearing of a single word is in doubt. Amphiboly sometimes results from faulty ellipsis or phrasal miscue. What sets it apart from other instances of these errors is that instead of being just awkward and momentarily confusing it is ambiguous and permanently confusing. Unlike Buridan's hypothetical ass, which starved to death between two baskets of equally appealing oats, the reader eventually seizes on one of the alternatives. It may be the wrong one.

> *The American Heart Association's recommendation for a sphygmomanometer cuff that is 20% wider than the diameter of the arm should not be abandoned on the basis of our clinical experience and experimental and theoretical considerations.
> *I believe this may happen in the next ten to fifteen years for a combination of reasons.

*To my knowledge they never arrived.
*In July Altman was joined as superior by Rodriguez.
*We are still seeking a perfectly safe agent that can reduce or stop
    the excretion of insoluble crystalloid material such as occurs
    when allopurinol is given.

The last sentence is an example of loose reference involving a subordinate clause of the *such* or *thus* type, a particularly common form of
amphiboly. "Make not oyour studies in haste, for in this way . . ." Can
you finish the sentence? Does *in this way* (= *thus*) refer to making your
studies in haste or to not making your studies in haste? Should the
sentence end "you but waste time and injure your mind" or "you will
attain wisdom"?
Amphiboly is especially frequent in negative statements.

*Biopsy alone can distinguish between chemical injury and idiopathic fibrosis. (Nothing but biopsy, or biopsy without other
    methods?)
*All oral digitalis preparations are not completely absorbed from the
    gastrointestinal tract. (none is completely absorbed, or some
    are and some are not?)
*Under these conditions the heart needs to pump less blood. (Must
    pump less, or need not pump so much?)
*The data prove no association between phenytoin and birth
    defects. (Do not prove any association, or prove lack of
*Return to the work environment may be attended by exacerbation
    of symptoms and decline in pulmonary function, particularly
    FEV_1; and the reverse is also true. (What is the reverse?)

A special instance of amphiboly is the **squinting modifier**, a word or
phrase that could refer to either what precedes it or what follows it.

*Lymphoblasts thus formed *more quickly* appear in the peripheral
    circulation.
*Changing drugs *frequently* leads to emergence of resistant strains.

ASYNTACTIC AND OVERLOADED PHRASES

The formation of compound expressions like *pacemaker, maturity-onset
diabetes* and *sinus impulse formation* is a special kind of ellipsis, which is
practiced more extensively in English thanin most other languages. We
may think of each of these composite terms as being derived from a

longer phrase by the omission of one or more connectives and by a shift in the order of the remaining words. Thus, *sinus impulse formation* is a more compact version of *formation of impulses in the sinus*. It is also slightly less clear, at least on first reading.

English is more daring, less consistent and less explicit than other languages in making compounds. For a notion of how vast and complex a subject this is, look over the pages devoted to it in the front of Webster's unabridged dictionary. Even a native speaker of English may be hard pressed to understand a compound that has been too rudely whittled out of a longer but more intelligible phrase. The composite phrase beckons irresistibly to the technical writer, who often falls for its compactness without noticing its obscurity.

The components of a **noun phrase** may be fused (*headache, gallbladder*), joined by a hyphen (*nail-biting, side-effect*) or left separate (*liver metastases*). In the last example it is a moot question whether *liver* is an adjective equivalent to *hepatic* or a transposed noun. In form, at least, it is indistinguishable from the noun *liver*. Most noun phrases follow the same pattern: *iron deficiency, suture removal, nerve section*. In a few cases, however, a prefix clearly distinguishes an adjective form which could not function as a noun: *multicenter study, preinfarction pain*.

Too often the technical writer succumbs to the temptation to replace a long phrase containing several prepositions with a dense aggregation of nouns. (See Schoenfeld R: Amazing Revelations! *Proc Roy Austral Chem Inst*, 41:298-299, 1974.) This device was first made popular by journalists, who found it so convenient and compact in headlines that they introduced it into their writing. *Iron deficiency anemia* and *plasma coagulation factors* can thus trace their ancestry to *wheat crop failure* and *record voter turnout*.

The meanings of these examples are sufficiently obvious. Confusion threatens when the noun chain is made too long (*Sample Drug Behavior Survey Instrument Design Section*) or when it is so overcharged with meaning that the relationships among its components are not immediately apparent (*guinea pig antibeef insulin antibody*). (See Gode A: Just words. *JAMA* 191:96, 1965.) The best cure for a confusing noun phrase is usually to translate it back into English, restoring the natural word order, replacing the stifled prepositions and perhaps converting a noun to a formal adjective. A phrase that cannot be restructured in normal syntax by this means is called asyntactic. Many asyntactic phrases are in common use in medicine, their meanings fixed by convention: *cold agglutinins, wedge pressure*. Newly fashioned ones, however, often mislead or confuse (*silicone clotting time*). (See Gode A: Just words. *JAMA* 198:132, 1966.)

Although the components of an **adjective phrase** are sometimes fused (*forthcoming, newborn*), more often they are joined by a hyphen (*space-occupying, burned-out, well-developed*). When the first member is obviously an adverb modifying the second, as in *richly vascularized tissue* and *more palatable vehicle*, the open construction (without hyphen) is safe.

It is probably immaterial to the people who live there whether Old Mill Road was named after an old mill or whether it is to be distinguished from another Mill Road of more recent origin. On the other hand, the advertiser of a *used lady's bicycle* would no doubt be indignant if anyone inquired which was used, the bicycle or the lady. The reader of a technical article needs to know whether a *small intestinal biopsy* is a small biopsy of the intestine or a biopsy of the small intestine and whether a *smooth muscle mass* is a smooth mass of muscle or a mass of smooth muscle.

The basic rule in writing is that every composite or phrasal adjective must be hyphenated unless its first member is obviously an adverb modifying the second or unless it is a stock expressioon (*iron deficiency anemia, medullary sponge kidney*). In *filtered-barcarbonate reabsorption, controlled-release tablets, small-cell lesions* and *small-intestinal biopsy*, the hyphen visually links the first member with the second and identifies them as parts of a composite adjective. In *plasma coagulation factors, smooth muscle mass* and *dense collagen network* the absence of a hyphen indicates that the first adjective modifies not the middle word but the final noun.

It might be objected that *filtered bicarbonate reabsorption* cannot be misinterpreted, sincer *filtered* could not conceivably modify the final noun. That may be true, but the reader does not know it until he has read the final noun. A hyphen between *filtered* and *bicarbonate* helps him to keep these two concepts together from the instant that he reads them.

A composite adjective that needs a hyphen in the attributive position (*dose-related response*) should have one in the predicate position also (*The response is dose-related*) unless it consists of an adverb and a participle (*well-nourished male*), in which case the predicate form is actually a passive verb (*the patient is well nourished*). Many style manuals exclude the hyphen from all composite predicate adjectives.

When one of the components of a phrasal adjective is itself a phrase, more than one hyphen may be needed to clarify relations.

buffy-coat-poor washed red cells
carbonic-anhydrase-catalyzed hydration of CO_2
a swine-influenza-like illness

This multiplication of hyphens goes against the modern editorial trend to omit them altogether from compounds. However, it is my strong opinion that if the writer insists upon inflicting headlines on his readers he owes them at least some basic traffic signs. Anyone who balks at my dual hyphenation still has the option of avoiding the need for it by writing good old-fashioned English.

Even hyphenation cannot quite bring sense and order to *non-English-speaking, noninsulin-secreting* and *nonsteroid-containing.* Of course, the writer or editor who is willing to overlook the difference between speaking no English and speaking non-English, between secreting no insulin and secreting noninsulin, and between containing no steroid and containing a nonsteroid will send such phrases to the printer with or without hyphens just as the mood strikes him. A more workmanlike course would be to remodel them so that their clarity does not depend on hyphens at all: "a relative who did not speak English," "a topical cream not containing steroid."

Many composite adjectives contain participles. Since, as noted in Chapter 5, a participle is never modified by an adjective, *ferrous-containing clay* and *viral-induced antibody* are ungrammatical. The only feasible correction of the first error is substitution of a noun: *iron-containing clay.* However, in the second case we can exchange either a noun (*virus-induced*) or an adverb (*virally induced*) for the offending adjective. The latter remedy can also be applied to the related blunder seen in *lymphocytic predominant Hodgkin's disease,* which turns out perfectly respectable when recast as *predominantly lymphocytic Hodgkin's disease.*

A typically, almost uniquely English practice is the use of a hyphenated verb phrase in an attributive position: a *would-be* pharmacist, *do-it-yourself* surgery, a *don't-you-wish-you-knew-what-I'm-going-to-do-next* leer. Though pithy and concise in speech, such irregularities do not belong in technical writing.

Less colloquial is the practice of transforming a prepositional phrase into an attributive modifier: *over-the-counter* analgesic, *in-home* use of paint removers containing methylene chloride, culture materials for *in-office* use, an *in-depth* investigation. This unidiomatic jargon, with its rancid savor of officialese and gobbledygook, is avoided by the sensible and conscientious writer.

Handling Latin phrases in this way (*in vitro studies, ex vivo preservation of organs*) is equally improper. Typically, as here, transposed Latin phrases are not even hyphenated. It should be unnecessary to sound a warning against such asyntactic horrors as *failure-to-thrive children.*

English contains some COMPOSITE VERBS of great antiquity and respectability. *Backbite,* the fusion of a verb with its object, and *fulfill,* which contains an incorporated adverb, both date from the Anglo-Saxon period (before 1150 A.D.). However, these words belong to what linguists call a closed group. Virtually all new coinages on these models must be considered at least slightly irregular. *To bloodsuck, to painstake* and *to earpiece* are not only repulsive but illegitimate.

Similarly, *to double ligate, to cardiac catheterize* and *to crisis intervene* violate English idiom. Like *to earpierce,* each of these Gothic monstrosities is derived by back-formation from a phrase containing a verbal noun and a modifier: *double ligation, cardiac catheterization, crisis intervention.* If we must have *to plantar-flex* and *to renal-biopsy,* let us at least insist on the hyphen as a small concession to intelligibility.

To clean void has an even more tortuous origin, from the adverb-participle phrase *clean-voided (urine).* Like *to roller-skate, to practice-teach, to baby-sit* and *to henpeck,* these composite verbs are asyntactic. No less hideous are babarisms like "Johnson is being on-the-job trained," which, though perfectly syntactic, follows the word order of German and Dutch rather than of English.

HYPALLAGE

We saw in the first chapter that in a purely isolating language like Chinese a word never has an assigned function, only a meaning. A Chinese word cannot be labeled as a verb until it is used as a verb in a sentence. Though English syntax is also chiefly isolating, we have many words whose form clearly shows their function: *cauterize* is evidently a verb, *retractor* a noun, *cancerous* an adjective.

This conventional link between structure and function is not absolute. In *discharge summary* the adjective *discharge* was originally a noun and retains the form of a noun, while the noun *summary* was originally an adjective and retains the form of an adjective. Still, the order of the words in the phrase tells us that it does not mean "summary discharge."

English can sometimes stretch the function of a word even further from conventional patterns, so that neither its form nor its pattern clearly shows its semantic bearing. A newspaper article about a disaster in Asia reports, "Inadequate food and untrained medical personnel are taking a harrowing toll in human life." If we remove the adjectives, we are left with the statement that the disaster victims are being killed by food and personnel. Though ostensibly these adjectives modify nouns, a little reflection shows that they do not really tell *what kind of* food and personnel the writer is talking about. It is not inadequate food that is killing people, but inadequacy of food; not untrained personnel, but their lack of training, or perhaps the lack of trained personnel.

This kind of syntactic transformation, known as hypallage (which rhymes with analogy), is not an error but a rhetorical figure. When Poe wrote in "The Raven," "Startled at the stillness broken by reply so aptly spoken," he meant of course that he was startled by the breaking of the stillness, not by the stillness itself.

This figure, common in colloquial usage ("I have had several sore throats") imparts vigor and concreteness to statements that might otherwise seem drably abstract. Unfortunately, such concreteness is achieved at the expense of linguistic truth. Though the meaning may sometimes, even usually, be obvious, the divergence from established patterns of usage and meaning is simple too flagrant an abuse of the tools of communication to be tolerated in technical writing.

I mentioned in Chapter 6 that the difference between a thing and an abstraction is not always observed in medicine. *Scleral icterus* is not quite identical with *icteric sclerae,* nor *nodal enlargement* with *enlarged nodes,* nor *flatfoot* with *flat feet.* Though in practice these pairs are virtually interchangeable, we cannot translate *preventing growth retardation in children* into *preventing growth-retarded children* unless we are content to equate stamping out disease with stamping out patients. The physician who confesses to *hearing absent breath sounds* may soon be found conversing with absent friends.

Illegitimate hypallage is such a common source of falsity and absurdity in medical writing that I now propose to barrage the reader with more than a dozen authentic specimens culled from the recent medical literature, so as to enhance his awareness of the fault and enable him to recognize it whenever he is about to commit it.

*The patient complained that the medicine caused *a dry* mouth. (dryness of the)

*Epidemic keratoconjunctivitis characteristically produces focal corneal infiltrates that can cause a transient, *mildly reduced* visual acuity. (mild reduction of)

*Immobility of sperm may be due to *missing* dynein arms. (absence of)

*In the Wenckebach phenomenon each impulse from the atrium takes progressively longer to pass through the AV node until one fails completely, causing *a dropped* ventricular beat. (the dropping of a)

*The higher mortality rate is almost certainly due to *delayed* diagnosis and *delayed* surgical intervention. (delay in)

*The problem in rhinitis is *too many* therapeutic options, not *too few.* (a surplus of . . . a shortage)
*Clinical confirmation of cardiac arrest depends on demonstration of *absent* pulses and *absent* heart sounds. (absence of)
*In phlebothrombosis the *sparse* inflammation facilitates the dislodgement of clots. (sparseness of)
*The physical sign of *an interrupted* reflex arc is *a diminished or absent* reflex. (interruption in a . . . diminution or absence of a)
*The patient complained of *no* assistance from the therapist. (lack of)

Most of these specimens follow the same scheme: an abstract or negative noun is concretized by being changed into an adjective, which is then appended to a more tangible noun. Here are some variations of the pattern which are not so easily translated:

*In nerve repair, the greater the deficit to be overcome, *the greater the degree of poor* regeneration. (the poorer the)

We might as well say that the surgeon has a command of poor English or that he displays sloppy finesse.

*Aspirin administered regularly causes the patient less discomfort than sporadically administered doses. BETTER: Regular administration of aspirin spares the patient more discomfort. . . .
*Unilateral Absent Perfusion of the Lung BETTER: Nonperfusion of a Lung
*the recurrent stone former   BETTER: the patient subject to recurrent stone formation
*Assessment of the Patient *with Suspected* Endocarditis (Suspected of Having)
*He was under treatment *for a possible discoid lupus.* (for a skin condition, possibly discoid lupus)

The last two examples are reminiscent of the device in journalese whereby *allegation of assault* is translated into *an alleged assault,* and *a prisoner accused of rape* becomes *an accused rapist.*

Hypallage is just one of several liberties that poetic license can take with adjectives, albeit the commonest in scientific exposition. The medical writer is not often guilty of speaking by turns of *many long months* and *a few short months* in factual narrative. The following example of prolepsis (in which the adjective anticipates the outcome of the action shown by the verb) is no doubt the fruit of carelessness rather than of poetic fancy.

*In July, 1971, the patient underwent an uncomplicated cholecystec-
tomy.

WIDOWS AND ORPHANS

Modifiers, including adjectival and adverbial phrases and relative clauses, are obligate parasites, incapable of independent existence. *Hepatic, self-limited, at the level of the carina* and *into which these acids are converted* are pure abstractions which cannot touch the real world until they are appended to some noun or verb.

This is often more evident to the reader than to the writer. In full grasp of his material already, the writer may think that he is expressing himself clearly when he is only sketching in the outline of an idea without providing needed details and connections. It is not enough to put together in the same sentence two components such as "Incising the abscess under local anesthesia" and "approximately 10 ml of seropurulent material was expelled." The first component contains a **dangling participle,** *incising,* whose headword is nowhere in sight.

A dangling participle that begins a sentence is perhaps less common in technical writing than one which comes at the end.

*The patient failed to respond to repeated countershock, suggesting
depression of the myocardium by potassium overload.
*The rubber band ligature then sloughs and falls away, followed by
granulation and healing.

The participle in each of these examples has been forced into an anomalous adverbial role. In the first case, *suggesting* modifies neither *patient* nor *countershock* (the only substantives present) but *failed,* a verb. In the second, granulation and healing do not follow the ligature; *followed* modifies *sloughs* and *falls away*—again, verbs, not substantives.

The second component of the botched construction known as a **Siamese twin participle** invariably dangles.

*Fifteen of the patients could be *maintained using* oral sucrose and
electrolytes.
*This procedure is frequently *omitted resulting* in many errors in
diagnosis.
*A tentative formulation has been *reached based* on available
estimates of potency.

*overfilling is thus *eliminated enhancing* efficiency and patient acceptance.

Another variant is the **crosseyed participle.**

*In an effort to rid the blood of excess phenylalanine the body employs minor metabolic pathways, thereby resulting in the formation of abnormal end products including phenyl-pyruvic acid.

Since *thereby* refers to *pathways,* the latter cannot logically also be the headword of *resulting.* But neither is it reasonable to speak of the body as "resulting in the formation, etc." The fault here lies not so much in the syntax as in the choice of verbs. Omitting *thereby* leaves a mild case of dangling participle to offend the purist. A radical cure would be to supply a more suitable verb: ". . . employs minor metabolic pathways, thereby *generating* abnormal end products."

Though the dangling participle was freely tolerated in English until well into the eighteenth century, modern taste condemns it on both esthetic and grammatical grounds. The writer who is adept at the mechanics of his craft and in full command of his material will probably not often leave a participle dangling. Even when he does, the resulting construction is not likely to lead his reader completely astray. Most dangling participles are silly and ugly rather than ambiguous or obscure. However, any unattached modifier lends an air of untidiness and confusion to a sentence, and the typical dangling participle can be expected to slow down the most astute and alert reader. On no account should a dangling participle be permitted to open a sentence, as it does in this last example.

*Grasping the mass firmly and applying gentle traction, the patient screamed in pain.

Probably many participles are left dangling by mistaken analogy with one of the following constructions, all of which are legitimate.

CORRECTLY ASSIGNED PARTICIPLE: *Establishing* an artificial plane of cleavage, we inserted the modified laryngoscope and advanced it under direct vision. (*Establising* correctly modifies *we.*)

PARTICIPLE AS PREPOSITION: *According* to Pressin these tumors are usually not cystic. (A dangling participle legitimized by long usage.)

PARTICIPLE AS CONJUNCTION: *Considering* that the colon also receives motor fibers from the vagus, these results are not surprising. (Another dangling participle legitimized by centuries of use as a connective.)

PARTICIPIAL ABSOLUTE: With the B-mode scan the images are recorded as dots, the size of the dots *being* proportional to the strength of the echoes and their position *being* related to the position of the transducer on the skin.

PARTICIPLE IN APPOSITION: The polyps, *being* highly vascular, were not excised until their pedicles had been clamped.

ELLIPTICAL CLAUSE: While [he was] *preparing* the formula Karns noted a curious acrid odor.

GERUND: *Correcting* these deificiencies will not guarantee a complete return of function.

The last two constructions conveniently introduce the subject of **dangling gerund**. Though a gerund is not a modifier, it can be said to dangle when its relation to the other elements of the sentence is not immediately clear. The following illustration is strikingly reminiscent of a dangling participle.

*On catheterizing the auditory tube, the patient obtained immediate relief.

In centuries past a gerund was not permitted to take an object in this way. One has formerly compelled to write *on the catheterizing of the auditory tube*. Our shorter form is less cumbersome but inevitably it gets confused with an elliptical clause, to which it bears so close a resemblance: *while [I was] catheterizing the auditory tube*. The only tangible difference is that the clause is introduced by a conjunction (*while*) and the gerund by a preposition (*on*).

In neither of these phrases—*on catheterizing the tube, while catheter-* grammatically a gerund has no subject, it is understood that catheterizing the auditory tube does not take place without human agency. Similarly, in the infinitive construction "to catheterize the auditory tube" some agent subject is implicit.

A gerund, an infinitive or an elliptical clause "dangles" when its subject is different from that of the main verb.

GERUND: *Porcine xenografts are applied immediately after *cleaning* the wound.

*The pectineus muscle can be exposed after *having identified* the femoral triangle.

*by *decreasing* the number of available protons, acidosis will resolve through a respiratory mechanism.

ELLIPTICAL CLAUSE: *The hemorrhoidal veins swell slightly when *standing* or *straining.*

INFINITIVE: *to open* a midpalmar abscess the incision is made at or slightly proximal to the distal palmar crease.

The subject of a gerund will nearly always be different from that of the main verb in nonparallel constructions like the first and second examples above, where the gerund is active and the main verb passive. The disparity of subjects is particularly evident when, as in the third example, the gerund is transitive and the main verb intransitive.

Dangling gerund, dangling infinitive and dangling elliptical clause are not so much grammatical errors as stylistic blemishes, and sometimes hardly even that. The examples of them that appear in passages quoted from Darwin and Osler earlier in the book are so benign that they escape the notice of the casual reader. At the other extreme are jarring grammatical incongruities like the following.

*By massaging the carotid sinus in atrial fibrillation, sinus rhythm will not occur.

This hideously lopsided way of saying that massaging the carotid sinus will not restore a sinus rhythm is structurally identical with the next example.

*By limiting the intake of alkaline-ash foods, the urine will not produce calcium phosphate stones.

Here, however, the meaning is that stone formation will be *prevented,* whereas in the previous sentence the same construction denoted the *failure of an intended or expected result.*

Such unruly babbling is the end result of tolerating the dangling gerund. A writer would be well advised to think of every sentence containing a dangling or discordant element as a warped plank: no matter which end he nails down first, the other will always spring and curl out of alignment, annoying and perhaps tripping the reader.

An **orphan relative clause,** one whose relative pronoun has no clearly perceived antecedent, is exactly equivalent to a dangling participle.

*This new soap is not powdery, which many surgeons do not like.
*Amidase cannot catalyze the reduction of arginine, which renders
   it ineffective.

In each of these examples the antecedent of *which* is not any single word
in the main clause but rather the entire clause. The objection to this kind
of construction is that it fails to make clear the link between the main
clause and the relative clause. Often, as in the cases above, the relative
clause is liable to be attached by the reader to the last word preceding it.

Even when a relative pronoun has a proper antecedent, the relative
clause can be so misplaced the the pronoun seems to belong to some
other antecedent. This may be compared to the squinting modifier and
various kinds of misplaced phrase discussed earlier in this chapter. In a
short sentence the fault may pass unnoticed: "He jests at scars that never
felt a wound." Moreover, there is no ambiguity in beginning a sentence,
"The senior author once removed a patient's gallbladder who . . ."
though the word order may generate amusement or irritation. In the
following example, however, the possibility of misunderstanding is so
great that revision is mandatory.

*It is assembled with isoleucine first instead of third, which is the
   usual arrangement.

The verb in a relative clause must agree with its subject in number.
Since *who, which* and *that* can be either singular or plural, choosing the
proper verb form requires a knowledge of the antecedent. Such knowledge was apparently not vouchsafed to the perpetrators of the following
sentences.

*Rarely, pulmonary emboli may be composed of nonblood constitu-
   ents such as fat, bone marrow, liver, amniotic fluid or tro-
   phoblastic tissue that embolizes to the lung. (constituents that
   embolize)
*It is the ingrowth of endothelial cells, vascular buds and primitive
   mesenchymal cells, which transform into fibroblasts, that
   accomplish wound repair. (it that *accomplishes*)

Pay close attention to the number of the verb in a restricting relative
clause introduced by *one of those which* or *who.* The antecedent of the
relative pronoun is not *one* but *those;* accordingly the verb in the relative
clause is plural, not singular.

*Acute enteritis is one of the benign viral infections of children that most often tends to occur in small outbreaks. (infections that *tend*)

A reminder is in order that a nonrestricting relative clause must always be set off by commas. The omission of these commas is becoming increasingly common in both journalism and technical writing.

*Laparoscopy permitted visualization of the gallbladder which was edematous and necrotic.

The omission of the needed comma implies that the patient had at least one other gallbladder, which was not edematous and necrotic.

FAULTY PUNCTUATION

The modern trend is to do away with as much punctuation as possible. The journalist, traditionally in the vanguard of language reform, now regards semicolons, hyphens, apostrophes and accent marks as superfluous splashes of ink. He uses the comma sparingly and erratically, and reserves the period for the solitary function of marking the end of a sentence, or of what he thinks is a sentence. The modern medical editor evidently labors under the delusion that *objective based curriculum, fifty years experience* and *eg* look more streamlined and sophisticated on the printed page than the established forms, and that this esthetic breakthrough excuses any diminution of clarity or readability.

Though some of the changes that have taken place in the practice of punctuation during the past fifty years have been salutary, others leave the reader lost amid a trackless verbal jungle. I have just discussed the comma with nonrestricting relative clause. Elsewhere I have shown how meaning may be jumbled by the omission of a comma ("from this point on the surface of the tongue is much rougher") or a hyphen ("The patient related artefacts in ultrasonography . . ."). The semicolon is moribund as a means of separating, while coordinating, two independent clauses.

Writing that is full of parentheses and dashes is also full of detours, backtrackings and tangential excursions. Generally it is poorly organized, and presents ideas out of their proper temporal or logical sequence. The dash is occasionally used to achieve a momentary and meretricious suspense in the assertion of a perfectly commonplace thought.

*A systolic murmur heard best in the second right intercostal space naturally suggests aortic valvular stenosis—but it is by no means peculiar to this condition.

When a word or phrase must be kept isolated from the rest of a sentence, parentheses are generally better than dashes. Even parentheses may be overworked by the writer who has fallen under the spell of the slick magazines.

*The role of digitalis (and other cardiac drugs) in her digestive complaints was not considered.
*Plaster casting of these fractures is neither necessary (nor desirable).

The sequestration of these phrases in parentheses, by which the writers meant to show that they are of subordinate importance, actually puts them into the spotlight. Moreover, by seeming to introduce a change of direction when in fact there is none, the device needlessly, interrupts the flow of ideas. In the second example *neither* clearly foreshadows *nor,* so that putting parentheses around the *nor* phrase as though it were an afterthought is a rather transparent device.

Do not use words and phrases in parentheses to make sense out of careless and awkward writing. When a pronoun is ambiguous unless followed by some explanatory tag in parentheses, there is no point in using it.

*He (Janos) felt that the board's postponement of his (Lee's) nomination was politically motivated.

Using quotation marks to highlight or emphasize a word or phrase is another amateurish trick avoided by careful writers. Quotation marks are not used with brand names in medical writing, or with formal technical terms borrowed from other disciplines.

*Vascular collapse is an ever-present threat and the means of combatting it must be available "immediately."
*Glues, adhesives, paints or resins that come in two separate containers are likely to be "epoxies." One substance is the epoxy resin and the other is a "hardener" or "curing" agent. In addition, there may be "modifiers," "plasticizers," and various "diluents" and "blends."

There is a spreading tendency nowadays to omit the apostrophe from plural genitives: *citizens band,* DOCTORS ENTRANCE. Even in formal writing we sometimes find a singular genitive that lacks the apostrophe.

>*For further information about dosage and precautions consult manufacturers literature.

The absence of any trace of the apostrophe in speech has perhaps contributed to this shift in usage. A century hence it will probably be the prevailing practice to form both singular and plural genitives with a simple *s* in English, as it presently is in the Scandinavian languages.

12

Faults of Concept and Style

Everyone has indulged, at some time, in the comfortable self-delusion, "I understand it perfectly but I just can't put it into words." Nothing exposes fuzzy concepts and wrong thinking so promptly and mercilessly as the attempt to express them in plain and succinct language. The careless or incompetent writer may, of course, choose jargon and circumlocution from other motives than the need to mask his confusion, but when a statement positively defies interpretation the reader cannot help wondering whether the writer has any clear notion of what he wants to say.

> *In hypotonic constipation the colon is usually partially full from one end to the other.
> *The external jugular lymph nodes, when not diseased, are small or even absent.

These are instances, on a small scale, of a class of foggy gibberish that is all too prevalent in medical writing. Such mindless babbling is far more injurious to communication than mere verbal inexactness. Many writers and editors who pride themselves on the conciseness and readability of their prose are remarkably negligent as to its meaning. As I observed in Chapter 6, accuracy in writing takes origin from accuracy in the writer's thoughts. One whose mind is undisciplined uses language in a haphazard and undisciplined manner, with the result that he loses control repeatedly of his material.

A careless shift from the collective interpretation of a term to a divisive interpretation, or vice-versa, is known to the logician as the fallacy of **composition and division.** A statement may be ambiguous if the writer fails to make clear whether a word is to be understood collectively or singly.

*Drugs of this class display predominantly nicotinic effects.

Though at first glance *predominantly* may look like a squinting modifier, no rearrangement of the words makes the sentence any clearer. If *predominantly* is taken to refer collectively to *drugs,* the meaning is that most of the drugs are nicotinic. If it is taken in a divisive sense, the meaning is that each drug is mainly nicotinic.

Colloquial usage often ignores the distinction between divisive and collective senses. We speak of a bottle of eye *drops,* and we say, "The three of them eat a *loaf* of bread at every meal." In many cases there is no practical distinction: "All sinuses communicate with the nasal cavity" means the same as "Each sinus communicates with the nasal cavity." In other cases the difference is profound: "Each glomerulus produces approximately 0.005 ml of filtrate hourly" cannot be converted into "All glomeruli produce approximately 0.005 ml of filtrate hourly."

Even when a speaker or writer neglects to draw such a distinction, the meaning may be transparent. If we hear that "A member of the house staff is present in the department 24 hours a day, seven days a week," we do not imagine that a single person has been incarcerated there. In the following examples, however, the failure to distinguish composite from divisive concepts is inexcusable. In the second and third sentences *both* is entirely superfluous, and in the last three it should be replaced with *either* or *each.*

*In the diagnosis of the acute abdomen, relatively few findings may indicate several conditions.
*Serum calcium can be divided into both free and bound fractions.
*Hold both feet in different positions.
*Urethritis may occur in both sexes.
*Place one drop in both eyes three times a day.
*Wrap both ankles with an elastic bandage.

This last may be just the thing for immobilizing a burglar until the police arrive but it can hardly be recommended as a therapeutic measure.

A **negative concept** is always abstract. A tumor and a murmur are real and tangible; absence of tumor and absence of murmur exist only in the mind. The privation of a quality, or of existence itself, is at best a difficult idea to grasp and transmit. In the last chapter we saw several instances of amphiboly and unjustifiable hypallage due to clumsy handling of negative concepts.

Introducing *no* or *not* into a sentence does not necessarily reverse its meaning completely. Sometimes the *not* overflows its bounds and means more than it actually says. "I do not advise surgery" really means "I advise against surgery." "It is not very important" means "It is very unimportant." "I didn't expect it to rupture" means "I expected it not to rupture." The rhetorical figure of litotes affirms a proposition by denying its opposite: "To ligate the artery without injuring the nerve is *no small* undertaking." But is a large undertaking really the diametric opposite of a small one, or, to borrow a comparison from benzene chemistry, do not the two stand in a meta rather than a para relation?

Language is forever finding ways to concretize negative terms by treating them as though they were positive and real.

> *Nothing was found in the stool, including ova and parasites.
> (How can *nothing* include something?)
> *No abdominal mass is generated de novo; it arises from previously normal tissue. (What is the antecedent of *it*?)

Another popular means of turning the abstractness of a negation to flesh and substance is expressing it obliquely. "He came to lunch in his underwear" means "He came to lunch without his shirt and trousers." When we say, "He has one eye," we mean, "He has *only* one eye," a usage reminiscent of the logician's drollery about the three-legged dog: "If every dog has four legs, and four is one more than three, than every dog has three legs." Whether this conclusion is true, or valid, depends on one's point of view. However, the obliquity of the following statements renders them false in any perspective.

> *Beriberi is caused by polished rice.
> *A water-soluble preparation is used to prevent lipid-inclusion keratitis.

Two other ways of expressing negation may be mentioned in passing. Both are based on the syntax of classical languages and have a discordant ring to the modern ear. "We found the palmaris longus tendon absent" sounds like nonsense unless we recognize it as an elliptical statement in indirect discourse, and supply the dropped words: "We found the palmaris longus tendon *to be* absent." Similarly, in "Use a clamp with the spring removed," *with* seems to have the opposite of its usual meaning until we realize that this is the nearest that English can come to an ablative absolute.

The concept of **risk,** hazard or danger implies not only the threat of some evil occurrence but the practical uncertainty whether such an occurrence will take place in a given instance. If a disease, drug or procedure *may be lethal,* then it *is dangerous.* To say, "Electroshock therapy may be hazardous," is to introduce an unwarranted degree of uncertainty. Either "Electroshock may be harmful" or "Electroshock is hazardous" restores the intended meaning.

A risk cannot be increased unless it already exists.

> *Venographic techniques in this day and age involve the use of flexible, atraumatic catheters and guide wires, and puncture procedures which need not increase the risk of thrombosis, phlebitis, bleeding, hematoma formation or other complications.

Since the complications mentioned arise directly from venography, the risk of their occuring in a patient not subjected to the procedure is nil. Admittedly thrombosis, phlebitis and so on can occur in one who has not undergone venography, but the writer has excluded such cases by his choice of the term *complications.* It is irrational to say that venography does not increase the risk of complications of venography.

VERBOSITY

In Chapter 8 I discussed conciseness as an aid to clarity, warning the medical writer not to let his sentences become clogged and clouded with amorphous sediment through careless lack of economy. Here I am concerned with exposing and decrying a turgid style of composition that deliberately multiplies words and syllables. This inane and irresponsible verbosity takes various forms, one of them being the compulsion to use **long words** when short ones would do just as well. Some writers habitually reach for terms that are too long, solemn and pretentious for the subject. Of two optional alternatives they always choose the longer (*orientate* over *orient, utilize* over *use*), and they will even dredge up illegitimate back-formations to gain a letter or a syllable: *sequestrate* for *sequester, dampen* for *damp.*

When the normal inclination to seek shorter, more streamlined terms is thus reversed, composition becomes a question of the survival of the fattest. A *one-drug tablet* emerges as a *single-entity formulation,* though how one can formulate a single ingredient is not clear. Here, as is often the case, the longer word brings with it fuzziness, abstractness and inexactness. Moreover, high-flown words like *sternutation* and *papyraceous* set a ludicrous and Micawberish tone.

The essence of verbosity, of course, is using **too many words**. Simple nouns and verbs expand into compounds and phrases. *Causative mechanism* does not really say more than *cause*, it just uses more ink and wastes the reader's time with five extra syllables. *Pregnancy onset* is the same as *conception, embolic phenomena* generally the same as *emboli*. *Shows* says as much as *is indicative of*, and *employed on a substitute basis* neither amplifies nor clarifies *substituted*.

No part of speech is immune to this senseless inflation.

ADVERBS: now → at the present time
  upward → in an upward direction
  therapeutically → from a therapeutic standpoint OR in terms
    of therapy
PREPOSITIONS: before → in advance of
  by → on the part of
  after surgery → in a postoperative type of situation
CONJUNCTIONS: and → in addition to
  because → in view of the fact that

In the last example, as in some of the others, we have more words but less meaning. Is the relation causal or casual? Is the "view" universal, particular, or perhaps unique to the writer? Is the "fact" established or only postulated?

Wordy and indirect constructions are an affront to the reader, since simple ones nearly always tell the story faster and better.

*The measurement of the patient's serum amylase level is the single
  most important determinant in the diagnosis of acute pancreatitis,
    despite the fact that a variety of nonpancreatic disorders also
    cause serum amylase values to rise.

Enlarging and encumbering a sentence with unneeded words can hardly fail to dilute and blur its meaning. If we excise the garbage from this run of English well-defiled, its essential message emerges at once with clarity, vigor and directness.

The serum amylase level is the most important clue to acute pancreatitis, though other disorders can also raise this level.

A surfeit of words can never produce a surfeit of clarity. Clarity increases as the quality of information given approaches the maximum that is needed, and then declines as further information is added. When, in revising your own work, you come across bloated, bleary sentences like the following, puncture and deflate them without mercy. Most of the obscurity will be found to have gone with the wind.

>*Even a mild former reaction to a particular drug justifies the recourse to some other therapeutic alternative. BETTER: A history of even a mild reaction justifies using a different drug.
>*It is obvious that ulcerative colitis and Crohn's disease are *two distinct and separable entities.* (are distinct)
>*He had been hospitalized *on six different occasions since the age of 13 years.* (six times since age 13)
>*Thyrotoxicosis *results in an enhanced sensitivity to the action of* endogenous catecholamines. (enhances sensitivity to)
>*A review of the literature does not *unequivocally support a definite predilection for the occurrence of spigelian hernias on one abdominal side.* (show that spigelian hernias are commoner on the right)
>*In mild diabetes, coffee *adversely affects the ability of the body to deal with blood sugar.* (impairs glucose tolerance)

Pedantry is a fertile source of prolixity. A pedant is one who makes a tasteless and unnecessary display of scholarship. When he takes pen in hand he cannot resist cluttering his sentences and insulting his readers by overstating the obvious.

>*The skin and nasal mucosa of each worker were examined by a dermatologist and an otorhinolaryngologist *respectively.*
>*Of 39 patients with documented staphylococcal endocarditis, only one-fourth had prior rheumatic disease; *the remainder did not.*
>*Digitalis-induced arrhythmias may change from one type to another in the same tracing *in the same patient.*
>*Intestinal obstruction may also result from adhesions produced during the course of an acute peritonitis *from which recovery has occurred.*
>*Lipogenesis has no relation to somatotype *and vice-versa.*

Specifying modifiers, which are sometimes essential for clarity, are heavily overworked by the pedant even when they add nothing: a *given* analysis, a *particular* procedure, the *individual* erythrocyte, the spleen *itself*, the cytoplasm *proper*, the patient *in question*.

A kindred impertinence is the proffering of self-evident alternatives.

*It may or *may not* be necessary to include the radial head in the fusion.

*The surgeon will usually have to individualize his or *her* technique according to circumstances.

Since the reader can easily supply the alternate words or ideas, the italicized material is redundant. *His* is a genderless possessive when used in a general or abstract context, and already includes the option *or her*. Similarly, *he* and *him* are equivalent to *a person* or *one* in settings where gender is of no consequence. (See Hussey HH: X-rated words. *JAMA* 235:64, 1976 and X-rated words: reprise. *JAMA* 235:1595, 1976.) By its frequent use of *and/or* and its predilection for phrases offering choices that are all the same thing (*for all intents and purposes, usual and customary, change or alteration, each and every, any and all*), a pedantic style reveals its kinship with legalese and officialese.

When a poet runs out of meaning before the end of a line he inserts a **cheville** (French, *plug*) to supply the requisite number of syllables. (It was Germany's greatest poet, Goethe, who remarked that poetry is all very well for those who have nothing to say.) The cheville is often resorted to by prose writers whose ears are better developed than their writing skills.

In Chapter 9 I tried to show that sound and meaning ought to be evenly distributed throughout a sentence. Some writers habitually put everything they have to say in the first half of a sentence and fill out the rest with padding. We are reminded of the peasant in the fable who always put a stone in one of his donkey's packs to balance the grain in the other.

The most prevalent form of prose cheville is a semantically inert word or phrase tacked on at the end of a sentence.

*A wrist vein is preferable to an antecubital vein *site*.

*The benefits of phophylactic antibiotics must outweigh the dangers of *antibiotic use*.

*The edema is usually dependent *in type*.

*Only this calcification shows where the pineal gland is *located*.

The final participle (*located*) in the last example may seem less boorish then the leftover preposition in "where the pineal gland is at," but it is still deadwood.

Sometimes the plug is completely overdone, so that long after the message has been gotten across the sentence goes rattling and rumbling on like an alarm clock that will not run down.

> *Once the diagnosis of tardy ulnar palsy has been made, therapy should be selected on the basis of the probable etiology of the particular patient's condition, whatever that proves on investigation to be.

GOBBLEDYGOOK

This apt and felicitous term, coined by Maury Maverick (see Maverick M: The case against "gobbledygook." *NY Times Mag* May 21, 1944 pp 11, 35, 36) denotes the style in which official government publications are typically written. Among traits common to gobbledygook and bad technical writing are abstractness, circumlocution and needless intricacy of syntax.

The almost exclusive use of the **passive voice** in medical writing to describe the actions of the physician is a relatively modern practice. Probably it has its roots in the same craving for objectivity and sophistication that begot the time-worn periphrasis, "A good time was had by all."

Though the patient and his ailments may still perform in the active voice, it would seem a shocking breach of decorum for a physician to publish such a statement as "I heard a murmur" or "We decided to try digitalis." Instead, a murmur *was heard*, a trial of digitalis *was made*.

The allegedly excessive use of the passive voice in technical writing is a favorite target for criticism by those whose tastes have been formed along more literary lines. The crux of this matter is that persons without technical training cannot fully understand technical writing no matter how well it is written. Instead of admitting ignorance they are apt to pick out the more obvious peculiarities of such writing and blame their lack of comprehension on them.

The passive voice is often the best way of expressing a thought, and sometimes it is virtually the only way, as when the doer of an action is unknown: "You are wanted on the telephone," "The autoclave is broken." As we saw in Chapter 8, the passive voice has a role in rhetoric, too. By making the receiver of an action the subject of a passive verb, we put that receiver into the fore-part of the sentence, which is where it belongs if it is the topical idea or rhetorical subject.

Useful and inescapable though it is, the passive voice ought not to be overworked. It tends to keep the reader at a distance, whereas an adroit writer tries to put him into the think of things as much as possible. Moreover, a passive construction may be a callow device for evading responsibility. "It is believed," "it is concluded," "it is recommended" seem unduly impersonal even when the believing, concluding or recommending is done by total strangers halfway around the world. But as substitutes for "I believe," "we conclude" or "the authors recommend" they are disingenuous and unbecoming. (See Gode A: Just words. *JAMA* 180:821, 1962.)

As I have observed more than once already, the use of language is a creative act and a form of self-expression. Every sentence that I utter or write is an autobiographical fragment, an embryonic statement of position or purpose. Though in formal exposition it is proper to curb somewhat this personal and individual element, to stifle it altogether is to be false to oneself, to sink into anonymity and nonentity.

Once committed to a passive construction, do not shift to the active voice within the same clause.

> *When the patient's position *has been so arranged* as *to expect* jugular venous pulse waves, the absence of such waves is a sign of venous obstruction.

As may be recalled from the previous chapter, *to expect* is here a dangling infinitive.

Noun-plague is the practice of replacing a strong and specific verb with a weak verb and a noun. *It hurts* become *it causes pain* or, worse, *it brings about a sensation of discomfort.* Not only does this style of composition impoverish and becloud every subject it takes up, but it also multiplies words needlessly.

> *In thyroid storm, impairment of liver function may *result in elevation of* [elevate] SGOT and LDH.
> *Gastric mucosal adaptation to continuous or interrupted high-dose aspirin regimens does not appear to occur. BETTER: The gastric mucosa apparently does not adapt . . .
> *Sudden cardiac *death* without evidence of acute myocardial infarction *is a well-recognized clinical entity.*

The italicized portion of the last example is an elaborate mutilation of *A patient may die.*

Adjective-plague converts an abstract noun to an adjective, which is then appended to a still more abstract noun.

*variability → the variable nature
*pruritus → the pruritic character
*bones → osseous structures
*seizure → convulsive episode

Gobbledygook makes its most extreme and deliberate retreat from the specific and the direct in its choice of terms. We may distinguish at least three classes of nuisance words favored by gobbledygook. **Jargon**, in one of its meanings, refers to the technical terminology of a craft, trade or profession. Gobbledygook typically prefers jargon to plainer and simpler words even when the simpler ones are in wider use.

Much of the jargon of medical gobbledygook consists of faddish inventions that have lost their bloom and unfortunately survive as tired clichés: *burgeoning diagnostic armamentarium, explore viable alternatives.* Abstruse and farfetched nonce-phrases like *individualized remediation, negative advocacy bias* and *maintain at thermal neutrality* [= *incubate at 37° C*] are less likely to endure than catchwords borrowed from commercialese (*initiate, innovate, finalize, time factor*), journalese (*sad commentary, profound implications*), federalese (*implement, facilitate, operationalize, decentralize, escalate*) and academic jargon (*awareness, involvement, expertise, dialog, quantify, holstic, symb[ol?]ology, typology, methodology, frame of reference*).

Another class of medical jargon comprises terms borrowed from other scientific disciplines, stripped of their original and specific meanings, and employed in a variety of vague connotations. Thus, the chemist's *aliquot* ("a volume contained in another an integral number of times") means, to the careless medical writer, *any measured quantity*. The mathematical term *parameter* ("a quantity which is constant in a particular case considered, but which varies in different cases") is applied in medicine to *any measurement whatever*. So, also *increment* ("an increase") means *any small amount*, and an *exponential increase* is *any rapid rise*.

Medical gobbledygook also relies heavily on **abstract words** of undulating and fugitive connotation borrowed from the general language. Nouns in this class include *approach, area, aspect, basis, case, channel, factor, feature, focus, issue, level, modality, perspective, phase, reality, resource, response, status* and *trend*. None of these is objectionable in itself, and each has its place in written English. However, its place is not often a technical paper ostensibly imparting concrete and specific information. Though we cannot stop to consider each of these words, let us take a careful look at one or two of them.

Why would any red-blooded writer want to call a method an approach? *Method* is straightforward, businesslike, confident of success. *Approach* fairly cringes with tentativeness and timidity. More to the point, an approach is *not* a method. Approaching a problem will not solve it; a method will. Approaching a patient does him no particular good; it is what you do after you reach him that counts.

The dictionary says that *aspect* means *look or appearance* ("a ferocious aspect") or *a view or part seen* ("the lateral aspect of the skull"). The first meaning is kicked entirely out of shape in "Practical aspects concerning combined live viral vaccines." Aspects of what? If of vaccines, what is the purport of *concerning*? The second meaning of *aspect*, familiar in anatomy, rests on the notion of looking at a structure, intact or dissected, gross or microscopic, from a certain direction. It has now come to mean any part, place or position whatever: "The azurophil granules are formed from the inner aspect of the Golgi apparatus at the progranulocyte stage." If we extend *aspect* to so broad and vague a range of connotations, what word are we to use when we want to convey the precise meaning of an anatomic view?

Nebulous verbs of which gobbledygook is inordinately fond include *achieve, constitute, deal with, determine, exist, indicate, involve, refer to, represent, stress* and *tend*. Especially frequent are such stereotyped phrases as *center around, in terms of, along the lines of, in essence, per se* and *is present* [= is].

> *The areas that we wish to deal with focus not so much on individual events but on great numbers of interacting factors.
> *Early recognition of maladaptive aspects of coping is an important clinical reality.

We may apply the literary critic's term PRECIOSITY to the euphemism and extravagance of medical gobbledygook. This is yet another species of circumlocution, another device for expanding sentences and blurring their meaning. Sometimes a general expression is substituted for a particular one: *pulmonary infection* for *pneumonia, eliminative functions* for *defecation, space-occupying* or *neoplastic lesion* for *carcinoma, acid-fast disease* for *tuberculosis*. A favorite technique is to replace an English word with a Latin one. Thus, *menstrual cycles* become *menses,* and the *genitourinary system, pelvic viscera*. If a Latin word is not available, an English one coined straight from the Latin is preferred to one of Anglo-Saxon origin: *pedicle* for *stump, inanition* for *fasting*.

Writing that is cast in this mold somehow manages to be unctuous and stuffy at the same time. At its worst, this stylistic mannerism imparts to technical prose the frigid pomposity of classical Greek drama. Preciosity is in particular favor among physicians who have been trained at the large Eastern centers. In many respects it resembles the false elegance and deliberate understatement of the British aristocracy, which in former decades were so studiously aped along the East Coast between Boston and Baltimore. For an intriguing study of upper-class talk (U-talk) see Ross A: U and non-U: an essay in sociological linguistics, in Mitford N (ed): *Noblesse Oblige*. New York, Harper & Brothers, 1956. See also Fadiman C: On the utility of U-talk, in *Any Number Can Play*. Cleveland, Ohio, World Publishing Company, 1957 and Ross A: *What Are U?* London, André Deutsch, Ltd, 1969.

Euphemism, paraphrase and all such beating around the bush are both unnecessary and unseemly in scientific writing. A haughty, mincing or affected style of technical exposition condemns itself to oblivion. It is a mistake to believe that the indiscrimate use of words typical of gobbledygook can add grace, strength and dignity to writing. It is almost as great a mistake to condemn every appearance of such words merely because they are commonly abused by shallow thinkers and incompetent writers.

The wanton **deviousness** of gobbledygook turns every sentence into a tiresome enigma compounded of equivocal hints and long tangles of words almost wholly devoid of meaning.

> *The ramifications of epidemiological and experimental research lead to the consideration of a multifactorial etiology for lung cancer in which tobacco could be a prime element.

Does *multifactorial etiology* mean that several causes must act together to bring about the result, or that the result may come about from any of several causes? Is a *prime element* an essential one, a statistically dominant one or just a relatively important one?

Gobbledygook can sneak up on a subject so furtively that it is past before we know it. The following was meant to be the topic sentence of a paragraph.

> *Possibly one of the most important aspects of any ongoing program is an evaluation that assists in developing a more effective process at a future date.

An assertion of fact can be so weakened with wishy-washy subjunctives and qualifications (*may be suggestive of, should often probably be considered preferable*) that it imparts more doubt than information. Many sentences of gobbledygook are the merest hollow platitudes, shadows without substance.

   *If indicated, the need for supportive measures must not be
      neglected.

This is not just too much of a bad thing—it is a sham and a fraud, a
staggering, whimpering nonsentence unfit for human consumption.

   Gobbledygook is a vicious habit that can take possesion of any writer
and thoroughly corrupt his faculty of verbal expression. Our daily observation affords plenty of evidence that persons who write gobbledygook soon come to talk and even think it as well. Its appeal to the inept
or heedless cribbler is irresistible because it is such impenetrable camou-
flage for ignorance and uncertainty. By rendering every statement tentative and equivocal, it greatly dilutes the author's responsibility. At the
same time, it lends a spurious color of scientific objectivity and detach-
ment.

   Some writers are so naive as to think that information served up in
this style will impress their peers. The writer who buries his meaning in a
thicket of jargon impresses no one but an imbecile, and is understood by
no one who does not already know the material. Furthermore, by es-
pousing gobbledygook as his customary mode of expression a writer
deprives his readers of the enormous range and fecundity of genuine
English, forcing them to accept a cheap imitation instead. A technical
paper conceived in this tortuous, inflated, artificial and repellent idiom
will come forth blighted and rachitic, if not stillborn.

   See Quiller-Couch A: *On the Art of Writing.* New York, GP Putnam's
Sons, 1916 (reissued, New York, Capricorn Books, 1961) Chapter V,
Interlude: On Jargon; Barzun J: The House of Intellect. New York,
Harper & Brothers, 1959, Chapter IX, The Language of Learning and
Pedantry; Reece L: Space-occupying gambits for medical writers. *JAMA*
200:56, 1967.

MEDICAL JOURNALESE

Acute undifferentiated journalese is the language of the daily newspapers, with its drunk and disorderly sentences, its surfeit of noun
phrases, dangling participles and orphan relative clauses, its scarcity of
punctuation, its fondness for catchwords and clichés, and its general air
of untidiness and confusion.

   *The meeting was marked by extra-tight security to prevent a repeti-
      tion of the guerilla raid on the ministerial meeting in Vienna in
      December and the abduction of most of the ministers, later
      freed in Algeria.

It is neither the writer's choice of words nor his syntax that offends us here, but his incoherence. Though his sentence hangs together grammatically, it is a conceptual hash.

The same kind of scatterbrained fumbling that characterizes newspaper writing has become one of the hallmarks of the ubiquitous throwaway, or controlled-circulation journal, the tabloid of medical journalism.

> *Direct observation of phagocytosis is a fascinating process to
> behold.
> *Self-examination would consist of regular palpation, early detec-
> tion of any change, and prompt medical attention if anything
> unusual is noted.

Since throwaways vary widely in style and content it would be unfair to tar them all with the same brush. The great majority, however, contain writing of extremely poor quality. I pass over in silence their offensively colloquial and patronizing language ("Another patient—let's call her Mrs. T . . ."), their lack of new or authoritative material and their generally low editorial standards. (See Greenwald AF: Give-away medical journals. *JAMA* 217:1705, 1971.)

It is perfectly obvious that physicians do not actually write what is published in throwaways. Material submitted by physicians is completely rewritten in a chatty, breezy, watered-down patter that combines elements of newspaper journalese and of slickese, the glib and facile gibberish of the slick newsmagazine. Many throwaway articles are generated by tape-recorded seminars or telephone interviews, the "authors" never putting pen to paper from first to last. Thus are explained such grotesque phonetic blunders as *normal tensive, normal glycemic* and *first* (for *pursed*) lips. Even when the nominal author has submitted a fully-developed manuscript, the actual composition of what appears in print is the work of a hack-writer with a degree in journalism, the intellectual resources of a bright ten-year-old and the literary taste of a Philistine. Since the medical knowledge of such scribblers is generally negligible, hopeless muddles like the following are by no means rare.

> *Little is known about the lesions caused by mumps other than that
> involvement of the testis can occur in the second week of the
> illness and may include gonadal involvement.

It is no part of my purpose to offer stylistic advice to the physician who is preparing to submit material to a throwaway, much less to show the editors of such publications the error of their ways. If, despite their shortcomings, the throwaways are more readable than learned journals, that is the learned journals' fault. Retribution comes when the throwaway style serves as a model of taste and correctness for contributors to the learned journals.

The most odious trait of this medical journalese is its flagrant and relentless abuse of language, its copious generation of sentences and even paragraphs of doubletalk, padding and sludge. Malapropisms, tangled metaphors and false generalizations lurk in every column, camouflaged beneath the glitter of smoothly plausible slickese. I know of no better way to alert the developing writer to these poisonous influences than to present and analyze a few examples.

> *Boutonnière deformity is pretty obvious at first sight but your task is not to let it happen by treating the predisposing laceration of the PIP joint.

No one who has come this far in the book should have any difficulty in recognizing three glaring syntactic faults in this sentence:

1. Inappropriate subordination. The obviousness of the lesion is not so related to the importance of preventing it as to justify the choice of the conjunction *but*.

2. Amphiboly. Negation is introduced in the wrong place. "Your task is not to let it happen" is a lethal mutation of "Your task is to prevent it." The result is

3. Phrasal miscue. The adverbial phrase following *happen* seems to belong to it rather than to *not . . . let:* "let it happen by treating."

> *Treponemal tests are used to confirm or rule out syphilis when the history and physical and flocculation testing defy a definitive answer.

Despite the jingle between *defy* and *definitive*, the reader is not likely to stumble over this sentence. The meaning is obvious—or is it? by *defy* the writer means *fail to provide*. The trouble is that nobody else means that by *defy*. Probably the writer had in mind some other expression like "The disease defies diagnosis," and carelessly blended two disparate ideas.

> *The risk-factor theory is laced with a systematic set of fallacies.

This is rubbish. To lace means to embellish, to adorn, to add a mere dash—originally, to add spirits or sugar to a beverage. Here the word is mauled beyond any correspondence to that meaning. Moreover, a *systematic set* implies both deliberation and method, which are incompatible with the notion of *fallacy = a mistake.*

>*Pathologic changes vary from interstitial edema to perivascular lymphocytic infiltration.

Here a scientifically naive copywriter gives us a choice between two pathologic changes as if they were opposite extremes rather than stages in a process. *Vary from* is fine in a description of hues in a flower garden or seasonal variations in temperature, but here it misrepresents the facts.

>*The exact mechanism by which propranolol exerts its antihypertensive effect is poorly understood.

As used here, *mechanism* is both a metaphor and an abstraction. Mechanisms are the work of man; they do not occur in nature. Though convention may justify using this word for a regular and predictable chain of biochemical reactions, calling such a mechanism *exact* is flirting with absurdity and drifting toward gibberish. The writer is deploring, however gently, the lack of *exact understanding* of the action of the drug. To soften the blow to the collective ego of the medical community he transfers the concept *exact* to the "mechanism." Then, instead of admitting that this "exact mechanism" is not understood, he says that it *is* understood—albeit "poorly."

>*As new techniques and treatments are developed, traditional concepts and approaches require closer scrutiny and justify repeated review.

Apart from a weakness for jargon (*concepts, approaches*) and a willingness to tolerate a hemiplegic comparison (closer than what?), this writer did well enough until he came to the last four words. Then his gears slipped and he made a semantic leap, leaving no tracks on the printed page by which the reader can follow him. "Traditional concepts and approaches," he tells us, "justify repeated review." I am willing to grant that they may *deserve* or *need* repeated review, but what *justifies* that review is the development of new knowledge and techniques.

The sentence which the writer gives us is an unstable mixture of ingredients from two others, both of which must have existed at least embryonically in his mind as he wrote:

As new techniques and treatments are developed, traditional
    concepts and approaches need closer scrutiny.
The development of new techniques and treatments justifies repeated
    review of traditional concepts and approaches.

Instead of writing both sentences, which was unthinkable, the author
made a rash experiment in hybridization.

Since the reader of scientific literature cannot stop and analyze every
sentence as I have analyzed these, he can be expected to swallow most
such statements whole, taking all words and phrases at face value. Even
if his intellectual integrity comes through this subtle poisoning intact, his
own faculty of communication may be damaged by its example.

It might be objected that I have been picking nits, and setting up
problems of straw for the amusement and satisfaction of demolishing
them, but a little reflection will show the justice of my criticisms. Either
a sentence means what it says or it does not. Either it establishes the
relation between two or more concepts with clarity, accuracy and precision, or it fails to do so. A sentence that does these things fulfills its
purpose, but one that does not is an impertinence and a lie; it has no
right to exist, much less to be published.

The predominantly negative tone of these last three chapters may
convey the impression that the practice of technical writing is largely a
matter of avoiding pitfalls. To adopt such a view is to ignore the
doughnut and concentrate on the hole. If you know your subject thoroughly, devote plenty of time to a preliminary organization, address the
reader with courtesy and candor, and then revise carefully and repeatedly
to eliminate inaccuracy, obscurity and redundancy, you cannot go far
wrong. The earnest and ambitious writer will aim just a little higher and
try to make his prose engaging and absorbing as well as clear and
correct.

Index